Intermittent Fasting
For Women Over 40

The Winning Formula To Lose Weight, Unlock Metabolism And Rejuvenate. Including many delicious recipies.

Kate Morrison

Index

Introduction

Women over 50 are the power of the world. From an emotional point of view, we are no longer as easily influenced by the negativity of the world as we were in our twenties, for example. We have embraced our strong, exuberant, and courageous personalities and no longer feel the need to apologize for our femininity. We have helped our families grow and supported our partners in their ambitions. We are at a time in our lives where we can celebrate who we are, and we have also learned the importance of taking care of our bodies.

Most women over 50 have most likely tried a variety of diets and are able to recognize that most diets that are in fashion for certain periods do more harm than good to their bodies in the long term. As we get older, our body chemistry changes, our energy needs change, and we must adapt to these changes to keep our weight in shape and protect our body from disease. The reason why trendy diets are never a good idea is because there is so little scientific research into the long-term effects they cause. No one really knows what happens inside a body more than 20 or 30 years later when the intake of certain foods is reduced. The key to maintaining our weight, increasing our vitality, and protecting our health is, therefore, to rely on a tried and tested method, used to centuries.

The concept of intermittent fasting is incredibly old. It is mentioned in some of the oldest texts and even the first healers had understood and recorded its benefits in the human body. Many cultures and religions have maintained the practice of intermittent fasting and even today some religious days are characterized by fasting.

The West, however, is now overwhelmed by the ease with which we can find food. We have supermarkets on every corner, take-away food, and ready meals in a few minutes that we just must put in the microwave. We no longer even need to leave our homes to have access to food thanks to the supermarkets and takeaway services that deliver directly to our address. As a result, we eat more than we need to, and we are convinced that the healthiest way to eat is to eat for the whole day.

Myths and legends about eating have been imprinted on our heads since childhood. At first, they kept saying "three meals a day!", then they told us that it was better to divide them into six small meals a day and, of course, there is the persistent saying that "breakfast is the most important meal of the day". We have become a company that continues to make small snacks throughout the day thinking that the more frequently we eat, the faster our body will work to burn the calories we eat. We have lost the value that fasting gives to our physical and mental health. Fortunately, however, there has been a revival of the intermittent fasting technique in recent years and the world has begun to recognize its benefits again.

As women over 40, we know very well that when it comes to our health, there is no one-size-fits-all option. We have awfully specific needs, and our bodies respond differently to various techniques to lose weight. You have probably tried different methods and perhaps you are discouraged because of their ineffectiveness and the side effects they have caused.

The Intermittent Fasting for Women Over 50 was written with you in mind specifically.

In this book we approach intermittent fasting not as a diet, but as a lifestyle that can help you achieve your weight loss goals without experiencing the yo-yo effect you probably experienced with other methods. In the following chapters, we will explain the concept of intermittent fasting and the science that supports it. The latter is something that tends to be missing in the explanations of other methods to lose weight, probably because there are no reliable scientific data and those few that there are do not always have positive results. This is one of the many reasons why intermittent fasting is different from all other dietary plans.

Among the points in favor of intermittent fasting, taken as a lifestyle, there is flexibility: you can adapt it to your needs and routine and there are several protocols to choose from.

We will explain all the different protocols in detail so that you can choose the option that best suits you. Instead of insisting you eat a specific menu and give you some vague details on how this plan works, we will make sure to give you practical advice on how to adapt the intermittent fasting to your life and how to keep it in the form of a lifestyle as you move forward. You can certainly use intermittent fasting as an occasional way to lose weight, but to benefit from all the improvements you can make, we strongly recommend that you choose to take this path permanently.

Intermittent fasting is also different from other diets and diet plans because the benefits are health related. Intermittent fasting also benefits your mental and emotional health. During the menopause, one of the biggest difficulties is just keeping at bay the sudden changes in mood due to hormonal imbalances, which can really affect our lives in a negative way, making us behave differently from normal. Fasting helps stabilize blood sugar and hormone levels so that we can be who we really are.

As with any new lifestyle, there will be some difficulties at first, but we will help you overcome them by approaching them in the right way and giving you many suggestions. Included in Intermittent Fasting for Women Over 50 there is a chapter with some tips on what foods are best suited to this path and some simple recipes that will help you bring intermittent fasting into the kitchen.

Age progression brings with it some problems, especially for women. It is thought that it is impossible to live a healthy and happy life and at the same time be satisfied at the table. Intermittent fasting is a journey that will lead you to have a great sense of vitality and well-being, even more than you imagine. Intermittent Fasting for Women Over 50 is the guide for this journey, and we look forward to accompanying you and helping you achieve your goals.

Here we are, are you ready to change radically? If the book will be to your liking, I invite you to release a review on the purchase site. For me Your opinion is fundamental!

Enjoy your reading.

Chapter 1: What is Intermittent Fasting?

You probably already know the term "fasting", maybe you have heard it in relation to religious practices or it is something you had to do before a blood sample or an operation. Most likely it creates in your head a hellish image in which people punish themselves for their sins. You may think that fasting means not eating. Intermittent fasting, however, has nothing to do with starvation or starvation. The term "starvation" implies that you do not have access to food and that you are, in some way, having negative effects from not eating. Going hungry is generally not a choice and is not under our control.

Instead, intermittent fasting means that although you have access to food, you choose when to eat and the experience does not harm your health in the same way.

Intermittent fasting includes assigning a pattern for eating at certain times predetermined.

You may be wondering how this is different from eating breakfast, lunch, and dinner at specific times. If you consider the fact that you do not usually eat at specific times but when you are hungry, you will have your answer. The two ideas are essentially different. When you practice intermittent fasting, you organize your day into fasting hours and hours when you can eat. There are several protocols based on timetables, which we will discuss later, through which you can assign different fasting periods and eating periods. The core of the idea, however, is that you assign your day a period in which you eat and a period in which you fast. Intermittent fasting is different from other eating plans because it does not determine what you can eat but rather when you should eat.

Intermittent fasting", in 2019, was the most popular diet in search engines with an increase of over 10000% since 2010 (Fung, 2020). One of the most popular intermittent fasting methods we can use to illustrate the concept is the 16:8 protocol. In this mode, you fast for sixteen hours and have a window of eight hours to eat. Considering that you don't eat while you sleep, so ideally, for at least eight hours, if you go to sleep at 8:00 p.m.

and wake up at 6:00 a.m., you should stay fasting until 2:00 p.m. Between 14:00 and 20:00 you can eat a light lunch and dinner at least two hours before going to sleep, to facilitate digestion.

This is the concept behind intermittent fasting, which alone will improve your health. If you decide you also want to lose weight, you will need to limit your calorie intake during the hours you have to eat and you will need to increase your physical activity. During fasting, you should not take food, but you can drink drinks that have few or no calories such as water, coffee, or tea, obviously without sugar or milk. You can take vitamins and supplements instead, but if possible, take them during the period when you can eat because, taken on an empty stomach, they could cause nausea.

Intermittent fasting is a natural way to organize our diet. Before we didn't have a constant supply of food, fasting was normal, and still today it is a natural process for many animals, some of which don't eat for weeks or even months while they are hibernating.

Our hunter-gatherer ancestors, after all, did not have the luxury of constant access to food, so fasting was not a choice for them; nevertheless, they were able to overcome very remarkable adverse conditions.

Our energy needs, of course, are quite different today from what they were at the time when we had to hunt for food. Sometimes we needed an immediate energy charge to overcome situations that occasionally arose. Today, our energy needs are more sustained, so it is logical that we should not fast for long periods of time.

In fact, we need a change of mentality to introduce intermittent fasting as a lifestyle since you probably grew up with the idea that having three big meals a day is the healthiest way to eat. We have also heard repeatedly phrases like "breakfast is the most important meal of the day", which is usually just a way to advertise sugar-rich cereal brands.

A lifestyle based on intermittent fasting has several health benefits, including weight loss, fat burning, stabilization of blood sugar levels, a limitation of diseases that can affect us, an increase in the cell repair process and increased longevity.

To explain what intermittent fasting is, you should also explain what it is not.

Intermittent fasting is not an excuse to eat everything within your visual range if you are hungry for the prescribed period. Any person who approaches intermittent fasting with this mentality is doing more harm than good to themselves. The basis of a proper lean diet-proteins, fruits and vegetables in quantity, fiber and fat-it doesn't change because you are establishing the time frame in which you can eat. If you hope to see all the benefits that intermittent fasting can offer, then maintaining a healthy diet and indulging in only the occasional glut is a must.

A negative effect of the sudden popularity of intermittent fasting is that there are people who consider it one of those fashionable diets and therefore give advice that is not good for your health. Learning the principles of fasting as a practice and how your body works when fasting is the key to not believing these deceptions. True intermittent fasting does not describe a condition under which you can eat as much as you want and what you want just because you then deprive yourself of food when you are fasting.

Another important factor to consider in understanding what intermittent fasting is is the period you fast. Avoid ingesting food during intermittent fasting should never be overly prolonged. There are protocols that require a 24-hour fast and this may be good for experts, but for beginners it is not recommended at all. Any period exceeding 24 hours is not recommended for anyone.

Intermittent fasting is quite flexible, the important thing is to stay true to the basic idea and make sure that what you are doing is improving our health.

If your goal is to lose weight, it is important to understand that intermittent fasting will help you lose weight relatively quickly, but in a healthy way. If you are not going to continue the intermittent fasting after losing weight, you may regain the weight you lost. You should at least strive to maintain a low-calorie intake and do more exercise to burn more calories.

This book gives you a great deal of information about intermittent fasting, but it is important to continue refreshing and recharging your memory. Make sure you choose your sources intelligently, though, and rely on experts in the field.

The best thing about intermittent fasting is that you will very quickly become an expert on the subject just by putting this lifestyle into practice. As you continue your journey, if you notice things happening to your body that weren't there before, do some research to see what process is causing it. This is how we learn about our bodies. Even at 40 years old we can learn body language and it is vital to be open to new possibilities.

Chapter 2: Science behind Intermittent Fasting

Most food plans avoid discussing science behind their methods because, in most cases, research is vague and contradictory. There is a significant risk in jumping from diet to diet to find something that works for you, and unfortunately this may only have a negative effect on your body in the future when it is already too late. It's really not worth it. Although it is important to keep your weight in shape, it is equally important to do it in a way that does not harm your body. If you are looking for a particular diet to lose weight, make sure you do your research first. A study of just one group of people is not necessarily true research.

Likewise, evidence based solely on testimony is not enough. After all, you don't know these people and you don't know if they really lost "22 kg in a single day thanks to the Caramelized Popcorn diet" (if it's not obvious, there is no Caramelized Popcorn diet. If there was, we would already be following it!). The diet industry is just that, an industry, and industries exist to make money. Of course, it is possible to make money in an ethical way too, giving correct advice to people and watching them get real benefits, but the opposite is also possible in the same way.

Fortunately, this is not the case. Intermittent fasting brings with it not only hundreds of years of evidence of benefits, but also a significant amount of laboratory research and other reliable studies. The impact of intermittent fasting on specific areas of the body can also be measured and explained through scientific processes that are also confirmed by doctors and experts.

The genius of intermittent fasting lies in its simplicity. There are protocols and additions that can be included in intermittent fasting, but the scientific support of the underlying principles always remains. It is a tried and tested concept, with evidence dating back to the oldest books in history. Even today, many cultures and religions still practice fasting because it really brings benefits. If you are still not sure if you are a good candidate for intermittent fasting after reading Intermittent Fasting for Women Over 50, you should consult a professional to get his or her opinion. Sometimes it takes a face-to-face opinion to convince you that a certain thing is in your best interest.

But how exactly does fasting work?

What happens to your body when you fast intermittently?

When we eat, our body turns food into glucose. There is extraordinarily little room for glucose reserves, though, and so as soon as that limit is reached, the body starts to deposit the rest of the food in the form of fat. This fat production is called "de novo lipogenesis". The ability to store fat, unlike glucose, is unlimited, so if you continue to ingest food before using up all your glucose reserves, your body will continue to produce and store fat (Fung, 2016). While this happens inside our body, on the outside we feel an expansion of our waistline, we notice that our body becomes softer than usual and we feel a general feeling of rejection when we look in the mirror.

The science behind intermittent fasting starts with insulin levels. Insulin is a hormone produced by the pancreas that helps our body transform carbohydrates into glucose. Glucose is the energy source used by our body and what it uses to give us energy. Our body releases insulin as fast as we eat, so if we do not eat for a prolonged period, our insulin level drops. When this happens, our body first starts burning any glucose reserves as an energy source and then it will start burning fat, mostly triglycerides, as a form of energy. This is the stage we want to reach through intermittent fasting.

When we burn fat, our body becomes slimmer and we can lose weight. Triglyceride levels in the blood are also linked to cardiovascular disease, so the more we manage to reducing these levels naturally, the lower the risk of developing long-term cardiovascular disease.

This is crucial for women over 50 because cardiovascular disease is the leading cause of death at this age. Intermittent fasting also allows our gastrointestinal tract to rest and repair, which leads to a reduced chance of developing cancer or other diseases related to the gastrointestinal tract.

The time it takes for our body to reach the stage where it begins to burn fat as an energy source is different from person to person, but most research has identified it at 10 hours. If there were no more fat deposits in your body, which tends to happen after about 72 hours of zero calorie intake, your body would start burning protein as an energy source. This process starts in your muscles and then moves on to your organs. This is, of course, a stage that no one should reach because it would risk permanent damage. This process in which muscles are used as a source of energy is the reason why people who have serious eating disorders or who are suffering from hunger because they do not have a chance to have food appear lean.

The benefit of intermittent fasting is the ability to burn fat without damaging the muscles.

In women over 50, this is especially important because our bone system and our muscle system must remain strong.

When your body starts burning fat, it releases fatty acids called ketones into the bloodstream. Ketones promote brain health, and their presence is useful to prevent diseases and improve neural structures that we will discuss in detail in one of the following chapters.

Lowering the level of insulin in the blood when we are fasting results in an increase in growth hormone and norepinephrine. Increasing levels of growth hormone is important for women over 50 because levels of this hormone tend to drop with advancing age. Low levels of growth hormone can lead to an increase in adipose tissue and a reduction in muscle mass. Research shows that growth hormone also plays an important role in weight loss without sacrificing muscle. Norepinephrine is a neurotransmitter and stress hormone that, when released into the body, promotes improved metabolism. Essentially, our body is always in one of two states, either a state of satiety in which it produces glucose or fat, or a state of fasting in which it burns glucose and fat. If we continue to eat, we remain in a continuous state of satiety without ever burning our glucose and fat reserves and thus increase our body weight. This is what makes intermittent fasting such a natural lifestyle. Our bodies are designed to occasionally fast. On the contrary, our body is not designed to stay in a state of satiety all the time, so if we have a small snack every two hours, our body will never start burning energy deposits but will always use freshly ingested food as a primary source of energy. Another favorite process of fasting is autophagy.

Autophagy is a natural process in which the body breaks down damaged or diseased cells and uses that cellular material to produce new healthy cells. Fasting has been shown to increase the rate of autophagy and thus increase the benefits of autophagy. Fasting brings the cells into a mild state of stress which is beneficial for them, since it increases their resistance, and therefore they are less likely to get damaged or become sick cells. Most of the research in the laboratory concerning intermittent fasting were made on animals, but human participants are becoming more and more common. The actual results of intermittent fasting, however, speak for themselves. It is generally difficult to obtain FDA approval to conduct experiments on humans, which is why a significant number of animal experiments must be performed before they can be performed on humans.

How Intermittent Fasting Helps Minimize Menopausal Symptoms

As an introduction to the concept of menopause - it's amazing how many women don't really know what's going on in their bodies - we should briefly discuss the hormonal changes that take place within our bodies and how they affect body weight gain.

When we reach the age of 40 or 50, the levels of sex hormones in our bodies begin to decrease. Our uterus no longer produces hormones such as progesterone and estrogen and we stop releasing egg cells into our ovaries. This results in the cessation of menstruation. This is quite a long process, though, and so if you have missed just one menstrual cycle, it doesn't necessarily mean that you are about to enter menopause. Generally, experts estimate that if you haven't had your period in the last 12 months, you are most likely going into menopause. From a health point of view, it is important to remember that menopause is not the only reason why women skip a menstrual cycle. If the absence of menstruation is accompanied by pain, discomfort, or loss, you should consult a doctor to make sure everything is okay.

With menopause there are also side effects whose severity and intensity varies from person to person. Some women may experience only one side effect while others may experience all of them. It is a unique, individual, and very personal experience. These side effects include heat waves, mood changes, night sweats, decreased libido, increased risk of developing cardiovascular disease, metabolic changes, depression and/or anxiety. All these symptoms are caused by hormonal change. This can also lead to constipation and weight gain despite not eating more than normal. And the latter is precisely the symptom on which we will focus more in this book. During menopause we also become more resistant to insulin and our bodies struggle to process refined sugars and carbohydrates. This resistance to insulin results in fatigue and difficulty sleeping.

Therefore, intermittent fasting is the perfect solution to balance our insulin resistance which makes us more sensitive. This helps our body to digest food properly without depositing it in the form of fat.

From the point of view of mental health, menopause has a not inconsiderable impact.

We are at greater risk of developing depression, anxiety, mental confusion, and mental fatigue. Clinical studies in animals have shown that intermittent fasting, helping to remove and renew brain cells, helps to decrease confusion, and improve brain activity (Bhatia, 2019).

One important thing that is not sufficiently known and discussed by experts and women is that from 5 to 15 years before menopause, you may be in a phase called premenopausal. At this stage, estrogen and progesterone levels begin to decrease but are not yet so low as to affect the menstrual cycle. Although the two hormones mentioned above are important, there are three other hormones that begin to vary and can cause problems. These hormones are cortisol, insulin, and oxytocin. In the opposite process to what we have already explained, estrogen and progesterone levels affect insulin but in turn insulin affects estrogen and progesterone levels. This means that you can develop a certain sensitivity to insulin during the premenopausal as you would during the actual menopause.

With advancing age, we also see the stress hormone, cortisol, reach extremely high levels due to the state of constant stress in which we find ourselves. When cortisol levels rise, blood sugar levels also rise, and this leads to weight gain.

The third hormone affected during premenopausal is oxytocin, also known as the love hormone. It is released when we form an emotional bond with other people and helps us feel calm and less scared. Oxytocin is the hormone that opposes cortisol. If oxytocin increases, cortisol decreases immediately (Cabeca, n.d.).

Menopause can be a terrifying moment in a woman's life. It can be compared to puberty, from the point of view of the aesthetically changing body and the things that happen inside our body that we cannot understand, and this leads us to feel overwhelmed. If you can understand the chemical processes that cause your symptoms, you will realize that they are no longer as insurmountable as you thought. Hormone replacement therapy can still be a possibility for women who cannot get used to hormonal change naturally. But like anything related to our health, it is best to try as many non-invasive means as possible before relying on medication.

Intermittent fasting is an option to try before switching to hormone replacement therapy.

Weight loss in menopausal women

In 2012, a study compared weight loss in menopausal and post-menopausal women. Each of the two groups was assigned a dietary plan to be followed with the aim of scientists to document and compare the changes in aesthetics and metabolism. One group was asked to follow a dietary plan based on intermittent fasting and the other was asked to follow a normal dietary plan with a limited number of calories (the so-called "classic diet") to lose weight. The study then assigned a maintenance diet plan to prevent participants from regaining the weight lost. The scientists were then able to analyze the immediate effectiveness of the diet as well as the consequences after the experiment was completed.

The group assigned intermittent fasting showed significant weight loss, decreased body circumference, and decreased fat mass. There were also decreases in triglycerides and total cholesterol. There was also a stabilization of blood glucose levels (Arguin, 2012). In general, the results obtained from intermittent fasting were faster and longer lasting compared to a normal diet with calorie intake restrictions.

Our bodies, during menopause, tend to react differently to the diets they are subjected to to lose weight and it is therefore important to remain patient and continue with your plan. If you have tried intermittent fasting in the past and got great results but it was before you went into menopause, don't expect the same results this time. You will lose weight if you do what you must, but it may not be as fast as before. If you are fasting intermittently with a menopausal friend, don't compare your results to hers. We're all different and that's why it's important to have set goals so that you don't lose your motivation.

How else does Intermittent Fasting benefit women over 50?

Women, in general, have a higher life expectancy than men and with advancing age, regardless of our state of health, we may develop certain diseases including:

Breast cancer that arises when the cells that make up the breast undergo mutations and become cancerous. It is the most common type of cancer in women and over half of the women diagnosed with it are over 65. Intermittent fasting has been shown to reduce inflammation within the body. Inflammation is one of the precursors to cancer diagnosis. Autophagy also ensures the destruction of mutated cells before they become cancerous.

Osteoporosis is the result of a decrease in bone tissue. Bone tissue diminishes over the years because our body decreases the speed at which it renews cells, so we cannot replace the cells in the bone tissue as quickly as they are destroyed by osteoporosis. One in three women over 50 is affected by osteoporosis. Weight loss helps prevent further decrease in bone tissue and autophagy helps to decrease the rate of cell degradation.

In the United States, although the elderly makes up only 13% of the population, they also make up 25% of type 2 diabetes patients. Type 2 diabetes is one of the diseases that, in clinical trials, has decreased with intermittent fasting and in some cases has even regressed.

Arthritis is much more common in women over 50 than in men of any age. There are numerous causes for the onset of this disease, including an autoimmune response leading to osteoarthritis. Arthritis in overweight patients is more painful, so using intermittent fasting to lose weight could lead to decreased pain.

Depression is the most diagnosed disease among women between 41 and 59 years of age. This may have something to do with the hormonal changes caused by menopause which, again, could stabilize due to intermittent fasting.

When is Intermittent Fasting not suitable for you?

From the very beginning, it is important to note that if you have had an unhealthy relationship with food in the past that has led to eating disorders such as anorexia or bulimia, you should not try intermittent fasting. The process of determining when to eat and when not can easily bring an eating disorder to light. Pregnant or lactating women and women who are trying to get pregnant should not fast intermittently during these periods. If you are at an incredibly stressful stage of your life or have trouble sleeping, you should avoid starting intermittent fasting until you can get the situation under control. If you are underweight (a BMI below 18.5), you should not start this process.

If you recognize yourself in one of these conditions, you can embark on this intermittent fasting journey, but only after consulting an expert:

If you have type 1 or 2 diabetes

If you have high levels of uric acid or suffer from gout If you are taking medication

If you suffer from heart, liver, or kidney disease

In general, thanks to the flexibility of intermittent fasting, most protocols can coexist with daily stress, because if you happen to skip a day, you can always resume the next day, so instead of increasing your stress levels, you can reduce them by not always sticking to your plan.

When you must decide whether intermittent fasting is for you or not, be realistic and kind to yourself. It is certainly important to focus on your health, but if you think you are mentally unprepared to change your lifestyle, give yourself some time and set a date soon when you are ready to start.

Although intermittent fasting helps reduce symptoms and sometimes helps to heal certain illnesses, it is important to listen to your doctor if you already suffer from chronic or serious illnesses and do not start this process if your doctor does not agree. Health must always be your priority.

People in incredibly stressful jobs where their decisions are a matter of life or death - such as police officers, firefighters, paramedics, and emergency room doctors - should consider starting intermittent fasting while on vacation. This will help reduce any chance of emotional and cognitive adjustment that occurs in the first few days of fasting and could affect their work. Alternatively, people working in these areas may start intermittent fasting on their days off so that they fast when they are not working. Professional athletes should arrange the intermittent fasting plan with their nutritionists to make sure they have more energy when they need it. Hydration is also critical for athletes and should therefore be of primary importance.

This chapter has given you a significant amount of information about the science behind intermittent fasting. It is a lot to assimilate and it would be wise to reread this chapter at the end of the book to make sure you understand everything. The most important thing in any lifestyle is to understand how it works, so think about this chapter if you need to. Do more research if you want to, but always make sure you know what happens inside your body once you start fasting intermittently.

Chapter 3: Benefits of Intermittent Fasting in women over 50

Intermittent fasting benefits people of all ages, but there are specific benefits for women over 50. You can see improvements in lifestyle, physical fitness, emotional health, and cognitive skills. Being all individuals, each person will have different experiences and benefits from fasting. You will need to focus on lifestyle. It is normal to want to focus on the benefits of body weight, but it is important to keep in mind that losing weight, for example, is important, but no more than vitality and well-being.

Lifestyle benefits

The simplicity of intermittent fasting, compared to other diets, makes it probably the easiest protocol to follow to get the most health benefits. Often, the complexity of some diet plans can cause people to fail at the first hurdle because, although they think they know what they are doing, they don't. This leads people to punish themselves through food, thinking that it is the right way to lose weight, thus only achieving disappointing results. Intermittent fasting couldn't be easier - now you can eat, now you can't. Often, special diets can be extremely expensive. You must buy specific ingredients and eat food that you would not normally eat. Intermittent fasting is also different in this respect. It costs absolutely nothing and besides a decrease in calorie intake in case you want to lose weight and eat as healthy as possible, there are no rules on what to eat.

The intermittent fasting is flexible, so sometimes it allows you to eat the things you like best. What would life be without a sweet, occasionally chocolate or pizza? With intermittent fasting, you can eat these things without feeling guilty because when you fast, your body will burn that food. Of course, this doesn't mean eating in fast food all the time. You will still have to follow a healthy diet; but you won't have to weigh the food and calculate its calorie content every time.

If you have found a food plan that you like, such as the ketogenic diet, paleo diet or other such diets, you can incorporate it into your intermittent fasting. There is no better food plan than a combination of two different plans, you will surely get even better results. Intermittent fasting is a fantastic addition to other diet plans and takes nothing away from other diets (Fung, 2020).

For women over 50, getting used to menopause can mean a temporary change in their lifestyle. In more serious situations, menopause can lead to difficulties in social relationships, especially with the partner. Intermittent fasting can make a difference and can revolutionize your life.

Health benefits

People of all ages should pay attention to cardiovascular disease but especially women over 50 should pay attention to it. The main cause of death of women over 50 is precisely a cardiovascular disease, which is one of the many diseases related to the heart or arteries leading to the heart. This includes obstructions, damage, and deformities of structures. There are several risk factors that contribute to the onset of cardiovascular disease, including smoking, a sedentary lifestyle, genetics, and diet. The latter is the main contributor. The most important factor, when it comes to diet, is the type of protein intake and the type of fat consumed. It has been shown that proteins from plant foods such as beans and legumes are healthier than animal proteins. Among animal proteins, the best is those that come from a lean source, so chicken and fish are always the healthier alternative to red meat. The fat component of red meat is another risk factor for cardiovascular disease, as well as other sources of fat such as cooking oils and spreads. Saturated fats are those fats we want to avoid, and these include animal fats, lard, and tropical oils such as palm oil. Unsaturated fats, on the other hand, in small quantities are healthier. Some examples of unsaturated fats are avocados, nuts, olive oil and vegetable oils. When we eat large amounts of food, our body transforms excess food into triglycerides which, if they reach too high a level, contribute to the onset of cardiovascular disease. When we fast, our body uses triglycerides as a form of energy and therefore reduces the number of triglycerides in the blood and, consequently, also reduces the risk of developing cardiovascular diseases. In the previous chapter we discussed the impact of intermittent fasting on insulin levels. In the time window dedicated to eating, we experience an increase in insulin levels, and when we fast, these levels drop. This drop in insulin means that less food is deposited in the form of fat. In animal experiments, it was found that intermittent fasting can prevent and reverse type 2 diabetes. Another thing that happens when insulin levels drop is that the FOXO transcription factor, which positively affects the metabolism, becomes more active within the body. This process is also linked to longevity and healthy aging. Another non-contagious disease that seems to be affected by intermittent fasting is cancer. Growth factor 1 (IFG-1) is a hormone remarkably like insulin and its presence is known to be a marker for the development of cancer. IFG-1 levels are reduced when we fast intermittently. Women over 50 are twice as likely to develop breast cancer, for example, and risk factors for other cancers increase when women begin to undergo hormonal changes due to menopause. Intermittent fasting is therefore a valid preventive measure for the onset of cancer in women over 50. Increased cellular resistance in people who fast intermittently has been shown to result in a stronger immune system and generally a faster recovery. The process of making cells more resistant through intermittent fasting is like muscle training. The more regular the training is, with rest periods in between, the stronger the muscles become. The process of autophagy that begins with intermittent fasting has been shown to help reduce inflammation in the body as well as oxidative stress, which is responsible for damaging body cells. Inflammation in various parts of the body is the precursor that leads to the diagnosis of many non-contagious diseases. The diagnosis of a non-contagious disease is much more common in women over 50 than in any other age group. For this reason, it is important for women of this age to use intermittent fasting and autophagy as a preventive measure for the development of certain non-contagious diseases. The cycle circadian is the name given to the rhythm created in our body by light and darkness (day and night). This natural rhythm controls our need to sleep and eat and has a significant impact on our metabolism, cognitive functions, and emotional health. It is our internal clock and if disturbed, it can have devastating effects on our body. It has been shown that intermittent fasting helps regulate the circadian cycle and, if it is out of rhythm, brings it back to its natural state. From an evolutionary point of view, our bodies are programmed to eat during the day and not eat at night. This, of course, is the opposite of some nocturnal mammals that have evolved and reset the circadian cycle due to the availability of prey during the night. As modern men, we have destroyed the circadian cycle by not going to sleep when the sun sets and continuing to eat during the evening. This affects our metabolism and our sleep-wake cycle, leading us to get fat and have sleep disorders such as insomnia. By using intermittent fasting to reset our biological clock, we can promote weight loss by optimizing our metabolism and getting more rest at night. In women over 50, this is particularly beneficial. As we get older, sleep disorders become more common. We feel tired earlier than usual, have restless sleep and can no longer sleep the same number of hours as before. This sleep disorder obviously has a significant impact on both our physical and mental health. The reason for this change in the sleep-wake rhythm is due to the decreasing levels of growth hormone in our body caused by aging. As we know, intermittent fasting promotes an increase in growth hormone levels, and this allows us to return to a more regular sleep-wake rhythm. It is important to emphasize that your last meal of the day should be eaten at least two hours before going to sleep and should be satisfying but not overly consistent. If you eat too early in the day compared to the time you go to sleep, you may experience hunger attacks while you sleep that would disturb your sleep. If you eat too much before bedtime, your body will still be disturbed by increased blood flow to your stomach due to digestion of its contents, and again, this could disturb your sleep. The importance of a balanced sleep-wake rhythm should not be underestimated because bad sleep has been linked to the onset of certain types of cancer. In addition, intermittent fasting has been shown to help regulate genes that promote liver health and balance the number of bacteria in the intestine. Intestinal bacteria play an important role in our immune system and it is vital to keep them in shape to support our immune defenses (Kresser, 2019).

Benefits on cognitive functions

As the years go by, especially after you turn 50, your brain's health starts to be different from what it used to be, and this affects your cognitive functions. The older you get, the more your brain, due to a spontaneous and natural process, shrinks and, although it is not something we can avoid, it is certainly something we can delay and slow down. From the point of view of intermittent fasting, the process of autophagy, which increases during fasting, can help remove damaged brain cells and use that cellular material to produce new brain cells. This process can alleviate the spontaneous process of brain shrinkage. The release of ketones due to the process in which fat is burned during fasting is also beneficial for the health of your brain. Increased ketone levels help protect your brain from seizures, Alzheimer's, and other neurodegenerative diseases. Obviously, as we age, we are much more at risk of developing neurodegenerative diseases. Diseases such as Alzheimer's and other forms of dementia have a wide range of risk factors including genetics and smoking. Fasting to promote autophagy and ketone production is one way to try to defend ourselves against these diseases.

A study of participants over 50, all with impaired cognitive function, showed that by increasing ketone levels in participants, cognitive function could improve within six weeks. It is thought that the reason why ketones are so important for cognitive function is because they activate the release of brain neurotrophic factor (BDNF). The brain neurotrophic factor helps to strengthen the nerve connections in our brain, which are the pathways used by the brain to transmit information, thoughts, and commands. Other studies have also shown that intermittent fasting promotes the growth of new nerve cells within the brain. Intermittent fasting also helps to improve neuroplasticity, which is the brain's spontaneous ability to create new neural pathways. This is essential to learn new things as well as to forget old habits. When we leave bad habits behind, we help the brain to remove an old neural pathway in favor of creating a new one. Studies have shown that intermittent fasting speeds up the healing process in people who have suffered brain injury.

Emotional Health

The positive impact that intermittent fasting has on the circadian cycle also has a positive effect on our emotional health. Older adults who suffer from sleep disorders are at risk of developing depression, anxiety, and other emotional disorders. Mood is also affected by sleep, and a lack of rest can cause irritability and unhappiness even in healthy people. When we practice intermittent fasting, we take the weight of pressure off our shoulders, we no longer need to constantly worry about what to eat, when and how to organize our day around it. Until you embark on the journey of intermittent fasting, you will not realize how much time you tend to spend thinking about food. When you can remove this pressure with intermittent fasting because you will know exactly when you are eating and when you are not eating, you will feel freer.

Intermittent fasting is extremely helpful in keeping your mood high with the bonus of feeling satisfied and fulfilled when you can follow your new lifestyle to the letter because it is much easier to maintain than other diets.

When we enter menopause, the risk of developing anxiety and depression increases, as do sudden mood swings, things that may be completely unrelated to us. Not being able to keep your emotions under control, suddenly, after most of our lives have been stable, can be terrifying. Intermittent fasting stabilizes the levels of hormones in the blood and brings emotions back under our control.

The emotional impact that menopause has on us is significant, and although intermittent fasting is a great help, it is important to keep in mind that sometimes we still need help living with the depression or anxiety that comes with menopause. If you've suffered from emotional disorders in the past, it's a good idea to discuss your options with a medical professional as soon as you begin to feel the first symptoms of menopause.

This is even if you are already taking antidepressants or other medications because hormonal imbalance can inhibit their effectiveness. Our mental health is also crucial to our physical health and it is therefore especially important not to underestimate it at this time in our lives. In the past, you have probably suppressed your emotions to help others. As women, this is a common behavior. But we cannot help others if we ourselves are in trouble, so it is important to understand that we are our own priority and we must make sure that we have all the help we can to live life in the best way.

In this chapter, we discussed the lifestyle, physical health, cognitive functions, and mental and emotional health that benefit from intermittent fasting. You will be surprised to see the positive impact fasting has on our bodies and lives. Understanding these benefits is a great way to motivate yourself. After you begin your journey into this world, you will begin to see these improvements and we recommend that you return to this chapter to compare how many and which of those benefits you are experiencing through intermittent fasting.

Chapter 4: Intermittent Fasting Protocols

Among the advantages of intermittent fasting, there is also that of flexibility. The basic dynamic is that you have a part of your day where you can eat and a part where you must fast, but the way you divide the day is absolutely your choice. Depending on your lifestyle, the structure of your family and work commitments, you can decide how to organize fasting by taking as an example several available protocols that you can also slightly modify to make them more convenient for you. Ideally, you should try more than one protocol at the beginning so that you can make the best choice. It is an extremely subjective decision based on what you think will give you the best results. The protocols we will discuss in this chapter have a dual nature. They follow the principle behind intermittent fasting: fast and then choose to eat what you usually eat but reduce your calorie intake to lose weight and maintain a healthy diet. Some protocols have been chosen by fitness experts who have modified them a bit. It is our intention to give you all the information possible so that you can choose the protocol that best suits you.

The 16:8 protocol

We have briefly discussed this protocol before. The general idea is that the

The first number represents the hours you must fast while the second number represents the hours you must eat. This protocol is the most popular because it is the easiest to follow considering that we already sleep for eight hours. This method is especially recommended for obese people who need to lose weight and decrease their blood pressure quickly. It is also suitable for beginners who have just decided to start practicing intermittent fasting because it is the one to which you can adapt more easily. This protocol is also known as the Leangains protocol and was made famous by fitness expert Martin Berkhan. You can easily have two or three meals in the eight hours you can eat, but it is recommended to have a light lunch and then a more substantial dinner. Women tend to do better with not very prolonged fasting and for this reason, this protocol is ideal for women over 40. Many experts advise women to limit the fasting period to 14 or 15 hours (Gunnars, 2020). Obviously, this is a subjective choice and if you can maintain a healthy lifestyle and no known side effects, the length of the fast is completely up to you.

The 20:4 protocol

This protocol is also called the "Warrior Diet" and was created by fitness expert Ori Hofmekler. The protocol consists of 20 hours of fasting and four hours in which you can eat. The ideal would be to eat during the night and the meal should be a "party" after the "battle". Although the fasting period is exceptionally long, some versions allow small snacks to control hunger. Fruits and vegetables are allowed among the snacks, so, in fact, it is not a real fast. There is extraordinarily little scientific research for this protocol, and it is not recommended for those who have just started intermittent fasting. The Warrior Diet also moves away from the classic method of intermittent fasting because it gives precise indications on what to eat and what not to eat. In particular, the food eaten should be as similar as possible to how it is found in nature, awfully close to the principle of the Paleo diet. The other option with the 20:4 protocol is not to consider it from the point of view of the Warrior Diet but to see it only from the point of view of intermittent fasting. In other words, following only the expected times of fasting and eating. However, it makes sense to keep the meal in the evening as well, to be able to go to sleep a little later and start a new fast.

A whole day of fasting

As the name of this protocol suggests, the fasting period is 24 hours. This method is more than anything else just the principle behind several types of fasting. It can in fact be used in a fast of only two days a month or even two days a week. This method has been made famous by the Eat-Stop-Eat diet, in which two days a week are completely fasting. The 5:2 method, also called The Fast Diet, made famous by the English journalist Michael Mosley, consists of two days of fasting per week in which you cannot consume more than 600 calories. The 5:2 method is one of the few that needs a careful control on the number of calories taken and is therefore recommended above all to people who want to lose weight. The other five days of the week do not require a reduction in calorie intake but only a healthy and balanced diet. The alternating days method falls under this protocol and promotes fasting every other day of the week (Kresse, 2019). There are several versions of this method and some of them require a caloric intake of no more than 500 calories on fasting days.

Fasting 6:1

This protocol means that for 24 hours a week, you eat absolutely nothing. So, for example you could start the day with breakfast and then fast for 24 hours until the next breakfast. If you decide to follow this method, it is essential that you keep hydrated during the fasting day because you will not take any food. Other beverages than water is also allowed, provided they are free of calories.

Fasting derived from the ketogenic diet

This protocol combines the ketogenic diet (designed to get you into a faster ketosis state) and intermittent fasting. In this protocol, the hours are fixed, and you can only eat from 11:00 to 18:00. Fasting is slightly different from classic intermittent fasting because it imposes constraints on what you can eat-no to complex carbohydrates such as bread and pasta-and also the order in which you should eat certain groups of foods. It suggests eating vegetables first and then protein. Completely removing carbohydrates can cause mental confusion, so if you decide to try it, be incredibly careful, especially if you are new to intermittent fasting.

Spontaneous fasting

In this protocol, you essentially fast when you feel like it and when it is most convenient for you. Although the structure of this method is attractive, it departs from the principle behind the intermittent fasting. Simply put, the idea is to use intermittent fasting only when you feel like it. For example, if you are traveling and have no chance to eat or if you are too busy at work to have lunch (Gunnars, 2020). Not everyone agrees to include it in the protocols of intermittent fasting since it does not give a clear division between fasting and the possibility to eat. It is considered more an occasional skip of meals when you cannot eat. It is certainly possible to use this method as you would with others but without a precise plan. For example, it may happen that at 10 a.m., during the week, you find that you must deliver a job in advance and then decide that you don't have time to eat and fast until dinner at 8 a.m. You will surely get the benefits of not eating for a prolonged period if you don't eat food and only rely on calorie-free drinks. This protocol does not work, however, if you want to lose weight as you would need to be consistent with fasting. If you do not want to make fasting an integral part of your lifestyle, the question arises as to why you would want to fast at such times.

Growing Up Method

In this method, fasting is scheduled on alternate days (e.g., Monday, Wednesday, and Friday), and fasting on these days is 12 - 16 hours. It is recommended to start with 12 hours of fasting and gradually reach 16 hours.

This method is particularly useful if you work away from home and on weekends you are socially active and have meetings with friends and family because it gives you the opportunity to fast during the working week and enjoy your social relationships. However, you can also fast for shorter periods at weekends.

Choose a protocol

Choosing a protocol for intermittent fasting depends mainly on what your goals are. If you want to lose weight, it has been shown that the 16:8 method is the one with the best results; however, this could only be since it is the easiest to follow compared to other protocols. The latter is an especially important point to consider. If you want to lose weight, you must follow three rules:

Your calorie intake must be less than the calories you consume. In other words, there must be a calorie deficit.

You must include physical activity in your lifestyle. This is the best way to ensure a calorie deficit without drastically reducing the food you consume - eat less and burn more.

You need to be consistent. This is the foundation in every regime you follow to lose weight because there is no dietary plan in the world that allows you to lose weight in a few days without taking it back shortly afterwards.

Some intermittent fasting protocols will probably allow you to lose weight faster than others, but you will only maintain the weight you have achieved if you are consistent with your diet plan. Drastic weight loss in a short period of time is not healthy for anyone and certainly not for women over 50. Everyone is different, and even the difficulties in losing weight can be due to different reasons. For some, the problem is eating too much in the evening, just before going to sleep. Because of the natural slowdown in metabolism when we sleep and the fact that we are not burning calories, eating substantial meals at dinner, or having midnight snacks can make us gain weight.

You can change protocol at any time because nothing is carved in stone. Choose a plan that you think you can follow and that suits your lifestyle. Start slow and increase the difficulty with time and experience. Not only will this give you a sense of satisfaction for completing short fasts at the beginning, but it will also help your body get used to the idea of fasting. This makes things easier and it is also easier to manage the side effects that arise in the early stages, such as headaches and constipation, which we will discuss in the next chapter.

Extended Fasting

Extended fasting is one of the most discussed topics in the intermittent fasting community.

In short, a fast is considered extended if it exceeds 48 consecutive hours. Opinions and research on how healthy this method is are at odds with each other and so now it is only a choice of the individual based on how they feel and how long they can endure. It is possible that our aversion to this type of prolonged fasting is due to the common idea that we need to eat regularly and in large quantities to survive. In truth, if we stay hydrated, there is no problem if we fast for 48 hours. When we are sick with our stomach, we have nausea and we are without appetite, we stay quietly without eating and deciding to do it even when we are well is not quite different.

The general opinion is not to advise women over 50 to fast for so long if you are new to the world of intermittent fasting. If the individual has already fasted for prolonged periods of time, continuing to do so will probably not lead to negative effects.

If this is your first time fasting and if you are a woman over 50, it is important to gradually increase your fasting periods starting from 10 to 16 hours and increase your fasting time until you try the extended fasting method. Always check with your doctor before trying an extended fast and make sure you are taking vitamins and staying hydrated.

One of the biggest risks in extended fasting is re-feeding syndrome. This occurs when food is reintroduced into a body that has been without it for a long period of time. The re-feeding syndrome usually affects people who have not eaten for more than 14 days but it is a subjective experience and depends on their metabolism and body structure. You may therefore have the symptoms of re-feeding syndrome even if you have had shorter periods of fasting. Feeding syndrome causes a change in body fluids and minerals and can, if left untreated, lead to death. It is for this reason that people who have not had the opportunity to eat for a long time, including patients with eating disorders, are treated with the gradual re-integration of fluids and only then solid food.

If you are trying to follow extended fasting, it is interesting to note that hunger tends to recede after the second day without food. The general rule is that if you fast often, you will notice a reduction in appetite. This is since there is a pause in the cycle of insulin resistance and a reduction in insulin levels. Your body's response to these factors is to reduce appetite but maintain the same energy expenditure (Fung, 2016). This decrease in appetite is a chemical process that has nothing to do with reducing the size of your stomach. You have probably heard some people talk about shrinking and increasing stomach size; in fact, there is no scientific evidence to support the idea that your stomach will change size after it has stopped growing. The only way to reduce the shape of your stomach is surgery that is only done to severely obese people who cannot control their appetite. What really happens is that when your relationship with food changes, you undergo psychological changes and chemical changes within your body that are the root that controls eating. It has nothing to do with the size of your stomach. The reduction in appetite happens when hunger hormone levels change and can also be attributed to an emotional or psychological change in relation to food.

The longest period without eating in history is 362 days! Obviously, we do not recommend this and, on the contrary, we wonder how it is humanly possible. It is certainly a demonstration of man's ability to go without food for long periods. During a study done on extended fasting, participants were hospitalized too fast for 14 days. The subjects were all predominantly obese and had a need to eat urgent to lose weight for health reasons. In addition to seeing numerous improvements in health and weight loss after 14 days, many participants said they wanted to repeat the experiment.

In this chapter we have addressed all the intermittent fasting protocols that have emerged in recent years. Some of these are derivations of other protocols and include specific dietary plans that are not essential to intermittent fasting. It is advisable to try several protocols before deciding which one to follow. One method might work well enough for you, but another might be even more suitable. The important thing is to fast intermittently, the how is not essential, so you have a chance to try as many methods as you like before choosing the final one.

Chapter 5: Practical tips for Intermediate Fasting and how to overcome difficulties

Although intermittent fasting is one of the easiest food plans to follow, there are ways to make change even easier and overcome some of the difficulties associated with intermittent fasting. Knowing what these difficulties will be puts you in a position of power because you won't be caught off guard when they appear before you in the first few days of intermittent fasting. It is often useful to stay in touch with an expert in the field who can give you advice, help and tell you about his or her experience and how he or she dealt with the problems in the first few days. Social media is an especially useful way to do this, as there are support groups and forums that you can consult, so you can talk to other people who practice intermittent fasting. This kind of support can make a difference, especially if you are facing this change on your own. Having someone to ask questions and get answers is crucial. It is also extremely helpful to have people to support you - someone who is willing to motivate you in difficult times and celebrate with you once you have achieved your goals.

The plan for success and how to stay consistent

Once you get the rhythm, it will be easier to manage fasting. At the beginning, however, it is important to have a clear plan to achieve your goals. Once you have chosen the protocol that is right for you and your lifestyle, you need to plan it about a month in advance to see if there are days when this protocol can't work and make changes to the plan so that you can follow it on those days as well. For example, if you have chosen the 16:8 protocol and decided to practice it from Monday to Friday so you can be freer on the weekend, but you have a regular appointment on Friday at breakfast, instead of ignoring the fact that this is at odds with your lifestyle, try to organize yourself in advance to avoid making last-minute decisions. You could then decide to skip the fast on Friday and do it Monday through Thursday and then Saturday instead, or you could ask your friend to meet you for breakfast on Saturday instead of Friday. Although this might seem like just a small detail, it is extremely important. If you want to stay constant, your enemies will be the very things you have not planned. Likewise, consider your family. Do you usually have breakfast with your family in the morning? If so, you will have to find a way to explain to them that you are starting to follow a new lifestyle that will make you skip breakfast. If you are always preparing breakfast, this is a good opportunity to change your habits. Cereals and toast are extremely easy to prepare for anyone. If you feel the need to stay close to your family while they have breakfast, turn that moment into a way for you to exercise. Always plan. What will you do if a colleague or friend invites you to lunch at a time when you should be fasting? What if there is a colleague's birthday party, and during your fasting window, you find a delicious slice of chocolate cake in front of you? Having a solution to these kinds of problems will help you stay true to your intermittent fasting protocol and you'll feel more confident, feel in control of your life and be able to make the right choices in situations that come up suddenly because you've already planned them in advance. Many of these situations can be solved by sharing your plans with your family, close friends, and colleagues. If you are using intermittent fasting to lose weight, be sure to throw away the scale and start using the tape measure. In fact, in any weight loss effort, no matter what method you are using, you should never rely on the scale to track your progress. The scale may lie, maybe not intentionally, but it doesn't tell you anything you really want to know. You want to know how much fat you have lost. When you weigh yourself, you are also considering water and muscle. If you've increased your daily water intake, you're weighing all that water, and if you're toning your muscles, then you're including in your weight the muscles you've toned through exercise. The only way to really know what your progress is is to measure yourself. A diary, whether in a notebook or digital format, and a calendar are two great tools for those who practice intermittent fasting. Use your diary to write down your goals and the motivations that motivated you to begin this journey. When writing your goals, be sure to use the Specific Measurable Achievable Realistic Time-bound (SMART) criteria:

Specific: Write exactly what you want to achieve. Writing "I want to lose weight" is not enough. Rather write "I want to lose 5 kg", or better yet, to avoid the "I want to lose cm" scale.

Measurable: How are you going to determine how much progress you have made and how much you are missing to achieve your goals? You need to be able to measure your progress not only to change something if you need to, but also to celebrate your achievements.

Achievable: . Don't set goals that are impossible to achieve because by doing so you are only preparing yourself for failure and disappointment. Be kind and honest with yourself; you are already starting a journey that many people do not have the courage to make.

Realistic: Make sure you are realistic with yourself about your abilities, what foods you can eat and other restrictions you already have and what effect they might have on your goals. You don't have to be too demanding with you same but still you must go a little bit beyond yourself to get what you want.

Time-bound: This criterion goes hand in hand with measurability. You need to set a period within which you can achieve your goals to measure your progress more accurately.

Setting goals is important and will be the principles that motivate you to begin this journey into intermittent fasting. If losing weight is your main goal, then you will need to organize your goals around how many kg or cm you want to lose in each period. If your main goal is to reduce the symptoms of a disease, then you will need to organize your goals around which symptoms you want to reduce or which medication you want to reduce or eliminate for that disease. Setting SMART goals is important because they act as a balance that you need to keep in balance. You will have to push yourself to overcome certain limits and not stay in your comfort zone by setting goals so easy to achieve that it makes no sense to set them in the first place. But you also need to be realistic about your time, the situation you are in and your state of health.

Share your decision

Choosing to make intermittent fasting a lifestyle is your choice, but it will certainly have an impact on the lives of the people around you. When you decide to begin this journey, it is important to explain to these people exactly what you will do and why. Be prepared to receive adverse reactions or surprises. Don't let this demoralize you; you have done your research and are able to explain science behind intermittent fasting to these people if necessary. After all, it is your choice and you should only share your plan with people who, if they want to, can offer you their support, you do not do it to get their approval. Your family will be the most affected by your decision, but they will also receive the most benefits from your new lifestyle. Intermittent fasting will improve your mood and give you more energy. Its multiple beneficial effects should also be important for your family because they want you to be as healthy as possible. Ideally, your partner should also start practicing intermittent fasting with you because it will make things easier at home. If he or she is not ready or interested in intermittent fasting, however, don't let this discourage you. It is possible to successfully follow this new lifestyle even if the people living with you are not doing the same. Your closest friends will be the second group to be most touched by your new lifestyle but only if your interactions most often include food. Your colleagues will be the ones less touched by your decision, but if there is a habit of eating together at work, it will be important to share your plan with them as well. By including the people, you love and care about, you will be more motivated to stay constant because there will be other people following your path. At the end of the day, though, you're doing all this for your own good and you don't absolutely need the approval of others. Fortunately, if you are a woman over 50, you have probably already reached that stage in your life where you don't need to seek the approval of others and their opinions count for very little. If you find it difficult to find support from people in your life, use some online options such as support groups to find people who are willing to support you. It is likely that you will be able to achieve your goals without any support whatsoever external but it is still useful to have someone to talk to when you are insecure or doubtful about certain aspects of fasting or just to celebrate when you start making progress.

Plan your meals

By choosing intermittent fasting as your lifestyle, you've already taken a big weight off your shoulders because you've planned when you eat and eliminated at least one meal of the day. You can go even further and increase your chances of doing well by also planning your meals and preparing them in advance. This is especially important if you aspire to lose weight because you will need to keep your calorie intake under control. You won't have to prepare your meals long in advance - a week is more than enough. If you have, for example, decided to fast from Monday to Friday, take time on Sunday afternoons to plan meals for the following week. This is especially important for the first meal of the day. You will probably be hungry, but you won't have to eat a huge meal because it might make you feel too full and you might feel a little sick. Choose light foods for your first meal of the day such as a nutritious sandwich, piadina or salad with added protein. You still want to feel full enough to get to your next meal without stuffing yourself. In the last chapter, we'll give you some specific meal tips, but in general, the key is to significantly increase your intake of fruits and vegetables and include healthy proteins and some fats.

Doing physical activity during Intermittent Fasting

Exercise is not only important for a healthy lifestyle, but it is also essential for losing weight. If you are already doing sports activity, you can continue your routine during fasting. You don't have to eat before your workout because you'll still burn energy reserves including fat, which is ideal. However, this is a personal choice. If you feel a little week when you work out without eating first, you can move your exercise time to after your first meal of the day. This will limit your appetite and speed up your metabolism. Regardless of whether you decide to eat before you work out, you should always make sure you stay hydrated. Much of the water we consume comes from food, so it's much easier to risk dehydration during fasting workouts. You should also keep an eye on your sodium intake and make sure it is high enough because you will lose sodium through sweating during workouts. Physical activity for women over 40 should be structured according to their physical state level. If you have been an athlete or a person who has always been active throughout your life, then you will need to change almost nothing. If you start training with intermittent fasting, then, as a woman over 40, you will need to make some changes. Increased sporting activity in women over 40 has many benefits, not just that of losing weight. Exercise helps your body minimize the effects of menopause, especially hot flashes, joint pain, and sleep disorders. Abdominal fat is one of the main problems once you reach this age and there are targeted exercises for this area. The sports routine for a woman over 40 includes the following components:

- Stretching exercises

- Aerobic or cardiovascular exercises

- Exercises to tone and strengthen muscles

The reason we include these three types of exercises is to get different areas of your body working and to get the maximum health and weight loss benefits. Stretching exercises include yoga and pilates, which help strengthen your abdominal muscles and increase muscle flexibility. For women over 40, these types of exercises are essential because they help strengthen the joints. In addition, it helps decrease the possibility of injury during other types of exercises. Aerobic or cardiovascular exercises work the largest muscles in your body and help your cardiovascular system. These exercises include cycling, jogging, walking, and dancing. As a woman over 50, you may already start to suffer from joint weakness if you have not trained during your life. In this case, you may start by doing more stretching exercises and lighter cardio exercises such as swimming or cycling. Once your joints are strengthened, you can start doing other types of cardiovascular exercises such as jogging. It is important not to overdo cardio exercises if you are not already trained. The "talk test" is the best way to know if you are training at the right level. You should be able to carry on a conversation with ease while you train. If you find it difficult, you should reduce the intensity of the exercise until you are able to speak with ease and then gradually increase your level. Muscle strengthening exercises help tone and improve strength and posture and reduce the chance of back injury. Hand-held weights are the easiest way to do this type of workout at home. If you go to the gym instead, there will certainly be a wider choice of weights and machines. Start slowly, without overdoing it, because otherwise you might hurt yourself. Start with a weight that you can work with easily for eight reps and then increase your weight until you are able to do 12 reps at a time. The most correct way to train is to start at the lowest level and increase the difficulty over time. Once you have finished training you should feel invigorated and full of energy, not exhausted, weak or sick. Choose an exercise you like, and you will probably continue to do it. Just as with intermittent fasting, you should choose a method that works with your lifestyle and won't work harder than necessary. Choose a workout method that you can do anywhere or a gym that is not too far away to reach. The more effort required to accomplish your routine, the more likely you are to find excuses to avoid doing it. Classic exercise should not be your only option. You can increase your sporting activity by making small, different choices in your daily routine. Walk your dog more often, take the stairs instead of the elevator, park a little further away from the supermarket or office. Small changes like these can make all the difference. There are many ways to measure your progress in sport including pedometers (pedometers) that are already included in cell phones and watches (WebMD, n.d.). Even if your goal is not to lose weight, you still need to include sports activity in your regimen to get health results. If you don't want to burn calories, your workout may be less demanding. The important thing is to decrease sedentariness and you will notice improvements.

Water is your friend

Much of the water we ingest comes from food, so when we start eating less, we put ourselves at risk of dehydration. Luckily, there is an amazingly simple method for

to make up for this, all you need to do is drink more water. We should drink about eight glasses of water a day, but this can vary from person to person and depends on how much you train and the weather. When it's summer, we sweat more and therefore lose water at a higher speed, this leads us to drink more at this time of year. Water is beneficial not only because it keeps us hydrated but also because it is a vital part of multiple body processes and for the proper functioning of the organs. Drinking water while fasting also helps reduce hunger. It is a way to distract yourself if you are having difficulty following the fasting times imposed by the chosen protocol of intermittent fasting. If you are not a fan of natural water, you can make an infusion with lemon, lime, cucumber, or mint to make it more enjoyable. Buy a bottle with an infuser that you can use at home, however, because the infused water on the market contains other additives and has a not inconsiderable calorie content. Other drinks you can drink during periods of fasting are tea and coffee. You should not add sugar or milk to these drinks, but if you really can't drink them naturally you can add a very small amount of sugar or fat-free milk. Green tea is the best option to drink during fasting. It tastes good even without added sugar and is rich in antioxidants. Some argue that it is also possible to drink other drinks with zero calories during fasting. This is questionable because ideally, we should not drink this type of drink. The preservatives and additives in drinks make them a bad choice for anyone.

Less on the inside means less on the outside

You are wrong if you are thinking that we are referring to the number of calories. We are, in fact, referring to your bowel movements. It is an important consideration to make when we fast intermittently because it is not something, we usually expect you to program. If the way you eat changes, your bowel functions and therefore your bowel movements will also change. It may take some time for your body to get used to the new routine, and while you wait for this to happen, you may face a period of constipation. You can get through this by drinking more water and eating foods high in fiber. If this doesn't change things and you start to suffer from pain and swelling, a mild laxative is just what you need to get things back to normal. Magnesium supplements are especially useful for regulating bowel movements and have the added benefit of being important in the life of a woman over 50 because at this age you start having problems with your bones and muscles. As we get older, our bowel movements change and what is normal for one person may not be normal for another. Menopause can also cause constipation, so if you are starting your intermittent fasting journey now and are already having constipation problems due to menopause, be prepared to deal with these problems. The good news is that constipation due to intermittent fasting passes very quickly.

Headaches and other side effects

Headaches in the first few days of fasting are quite common. It is nothing to worry about because it is the body's natural reaction to changes in sodium in your body. This happens because of the change in diet. A small amount of salt and good hydration helps to reduce or minimize the severity of these headaches because the salt replaces the

electrolytes that can be the cause of head pain. Heartburn, dizziness, and muscle cramps may be other side effects of the first days of intermittent fasting. Dizziness can be caused by dehydration or low sodium content which can be improved by drinking a broth or mineral water. Dizziness may also be due to low blood pressure. Fasting helps to reduce your blood pressure, so if you are taking medication for hypertension (high blood pressure), then that further reduction can take your blood pressure to a too low level. If you think this is your problem, consult a doctor to see if you can reduce the dosage. Hypertension is quite common in women over

40 so the benefit of reducing blood pressure is very favourable. Heartburn can occur if the first meal of the day is particularly high. If, on the other hand, you eat a lighter meal and make sure you stay in an upright position for at least 30 minutes after eating (do not go to sleep immediately after lunch), you will reduce your chances of suffering from heartburn. As with the other side effects, this will disappear within a few days without external help. Muscle cramps are often caused by a lack of magnesium. You can fix this problem by starting to take magnesium supplements or taking a bath in Epsom salts.

Keep busy

Especially in the first days of fasting you will often find yourself thinking about food and this will lead you to think that you are hungrier than you really are. If, before you start fasting intermittently, you were inclined to eat out of boredom, this point will be especially important. Prepare activities in advance that will be able to distract you from the fact that you are not eating. It would be preferable to choose some remarkably interesting activities such as learning something new or starting projects that require a lot of attention. If you just watch TV or text with a friend, you will probably still have a lot of energy to think about food. This is another reason why, if you work away from home, you will find it easier to fast when you are at work. If you are focused on work, you are more likely to forget that you are fasting and get on with your day in a more relaxed way. The phrase "the power of the mind over the body" is very pertinent to the discourse of hunger. The waves of appetite pass and a little distraction, drinking water or meditating for a few minutes will help you get through them more quickly. Remember why you decided to start this journey. Think back to all the benefits fasting can give you. See yourself once you've received all those benefits - achieve your weight goal, have more energy, increase longevity, have a stronger immune system and a better mood. Surely, it's not worth risking all this for a small hunger attack. If it can help you, think about your family. Consider how, through fasting, you are increasing your chances of spending more time with them. Everyone has a different motivation that drives them to continue, find your own and cling to it. Hunger will pass. Remember that you can eat, just not at that precise moment. And remember that just because you're not physically eating food, it doesn't mean your body isn't "eating". On the contrary when you fast, your body feeds on your fat deposits (Fung, 2020). In this chapter, we have given you some tips and tricks on how to deal with the difficulties that may arise due to this change in your lifestyle. When compared to other weight loss diets, intermittent fasting is the one with the least side effects and those that are, are easy to overcome. It is essential to know that they will be there and prevent them so that you are not caught off guard at that moment.

Chapter 6: Foods suitable for Intermittent Fasting and some recipes

Although intermittent fasting does not dictate which foods you should eat and which you should not, there are certainly more appropriate foods. Since you are limiting your diet to a specific period, it is important to eat in a healthy and balanced way to avoid deficiencies in any nutritional group. The recipes that we have decided to include in this chapter have been selected precisely because they include foods that will help you on this path. We have also included the nutritional information of each recipe and the number of calories (if you want to lose weight), carbohydrates, fat, fiber, protein, and salt. Salt serves in our diet because it can act as an electrolyte, but it hurts if it is in excess, so it is important to consider how much salt is consumed daily. Keep in mind that there is sodium hidden in almost everything. We have also included a section in all the recipes where we tell you in advance if you need specific tools to make them. All these recipes may have alternatives so be sure to read the suggestions and possible variations at the end of each recipe to find out some ways to change the dish and make it more suitable for you.

Drinks

During your fasting period, water, coffee, and tea without additives are ideal for staying hydrated. Cinnamon tea and licorice tea have hunger-relieving properties that can help you if you get hungry. During the time you can eat, you can also drink other types of drinks, but always be careful about sugar levels in drinks on the market because even fruit juices contain a high amount of sugar and other additives. Coffee, if taken in moderation, is extremely healthy. It improves concentration and promotes healing of the liver if damaged.

Recommended foods during the hours you can eat

Foods rich in fiber make you feel fuller for longer. In addition, they help to counter the constipation that may arise in the first days of fasting. Some examples of foods rich in fiber are fruits, vegetables, nuts, and beans. Raspberries are also rich in fiber and can be a great snack. Lentils are another fiber-rich food and, in addition, are an excellent source of protein and iron. Cruciferous vegetables such as cauliflower, broccoli and Brussels sprouts contain a high fiber content. Protein-rich foods are great because they make you feel full for a longer period and are important if you are training your muscles. Some examples of protein-rich foods are tofu, fish, meat, legumes, and nuts. A healthy diet includes extraordinarily little red meat. Excessive consumption of red meat has been linked to the onset of many non-contagious diseases including cardiovascular disease, diabetes, and hypertension. If you are unable to completely remove animal protein from your diet (or prefer not to), try eating as little as possible. Chicken and fish are better options than red meat, while vegetable protein is the healthier option. A cup of protein contains about half the protein in a cup of red meat, so to get the same amount of protein, you'll need to double the portion. This It might seem like a problem, but with vegetable proteins it is not because they are rich in vitamins and minerals and it is worth eating an extra portion. Another excellent source of vegetable protein is seitan. It is known as "grain meat" and can be cooked the same way you would cook meat and has the same texture. Soy is an excellent source of isoflavones that inhibit cellular damage from the sun and promote anti-aging (certainly especially useful for women over 50!). Salmon is one of the healthiest sources of animal proteins because it contains a high number of Omega fatty acids, useful for women over 50 because they help the brain to stay healthy. Always choose wild caught salmon because the farmed salmon is full of antibiotics and is much less nutritious than the first one. If you are not following a diet that excludes carbohydrates, you have no reason to avoid them if you practice intermittent fasting. Integral sandwiches and piadine are extremely easy and quick options to prepare and a source of carbohydrates that you can digest quickly to get energy during your workouts. When potatoes get cold, they form a resistant layer of starch that contains prebiotics useful for bacteria in our intestines that play an important role in our immune system. Other examples of easy to digest carbohydrates are artichokes, apples, bananas, and asparagus. Sources of carbohydrate-free prebiotics are garlic, leeks, chard, and spinach. It is not uncommon for those who practice intermittent fasting to have calcium and vitamin D deficiency. The main reason is that both calcium and vitamin D are mainly found in dairy products and we eat this type of food more at breakfast. If we decide to skip breakfast for fasting, many of these dairy products are missing in our diet and consequently also vitamin D and calcium. This is not something that should push us to stop fasting intermittently because we just include these foods in our other meals. In addition to milk and milk products, black cabbage, tofu, and soya are excellent sources of calcium and vitamin D. Another component of dairy products that we may miss is vitamin K. Plums are rich in vitamin K as well as fiber. Vitamin K is essential for bone health, which is an area that becomes more and more important with aging. The fact that it also contains fiber is a bonus. Fats have a bad reputation that is not always deserved. A low-fat content is not always the best option, especially if the low-fat option contains saturated fat. We need fat in our diet, but we must pay attention to which fats we choose. To fry, you don't have to heat the oil until there is smoke because it creates carcinogenic (cancer-causing) properties. Clarified butter is the option that has the highest evaporation point. To keep your intestines healthy while you fast and avoid constipation due to menopause as a benefit, you must include probiotics, an important part of this regimen. The best sources are kefir, kombucha and sauerkraut. Yogurt can be a source of probiotics, but it depends on how it is produced.

Highly processed yogurts will have an exceptionally low number of probiotics, so it is easier to eat sources as pure as those mentioned above. Probiotic supplements are a possibility, but it is always better to try to supplement them with food first because it is the most effective method. Whole grains are a better option than refined cereals because the portion that is removed in the refining process is the most nutritious part. Whole grains also give a sense of greater satiety and contain more fiber. Some examples of whole grains include spelt, amaranth, millet, bulgur, and sorghum (Rizzo, 2018). Barley and oats contain beta-glucans, a type of fiber that helps control blood sugar levels. When blood sugar is stable, we are hungry less often. Maca grass is a superfood that is phenomenal in women over 40 as it regulates hormone levels and insulin and blood sugar levels. It is a tuber remarkably like the taste of radish and is originally from Peru. Maca is sold in powder form and can be included in smoothies, mixed in yoghurt, or dissolved in tea. A clinical study has been done on the positive effects of maca in menopausal women. Over a period of four months, a group of both premenopausal and menopausal women added two tablespoons of maca grass to their diet daily. All participants noticed a reduction in menopausal symptoms. The experiment also showed that their hormone levels had become much more stable than before (Cabecca, n.d.).

Recommended foods to interrupt fasting

When you must stop fasting, be careful not to eat too much. Not only will you feel sick, but you won't even be able to distribute the various meals you plan to eat during the time you are allowed to do so, and most likely this will lead you to be hungrier during the next fast. Always break the fasting window with a light, easily digestible meal so that your blood sugar level rises relatively quickly, and then have a more substantial meal later. By interrupting your fast with a light meal, you will be surprised at how easy it really is to keep hunger and satiation at bay. You don't need a huge plate of food to sustain you, even when you are fasting intermittently. Hummus is an excellent option to stop fasting. This chickpea puree sauce is delicious. Eat it with a cup of chopped vegetables for a healthy meal that sustains you through dinner. Hummus is also good spread on crackers or rye bread. Smoothies are another healthy option as a first meal after fasting. Fill your smoothies with as many fruits and vegetables as possible to increase your intake of antioxidants and vitamins. Use frozen fruits and vegetables to make things easier for you - they have the same number of vitamins. Blueberries are one of the best ingredients for smoothies because they are rich in antioxidants. Papaya contains papain which makes protein digestion faster. If you choose to make a protein-rich meal to break your fast, include a few pieces of papaya to help digestion. You can break your fast with a handful of nuts and dried fruits, or you can eat them before training as a protein source. Studies have shown that people who eat nuts regularly reduce the risk of developing cardiovascular disease and type 2 diabetes (Weeks, 2019). Almonds and walnuts are particularly good when added to salad or pasta. Peanut butter (preferably without added sugar) is another suitable alternative to stop fasting. Avocado in salad or on a slice of wholemeal bread is a great way to break the fast and is also a light and nutritious meal. Avocado is a source of unsaturated fat and is very filling. When you add half an avocado to your lunch, you'll be full for more hours than when you don't. You can also slice the avocado and eat it with a hard-boiled egg that is a great source of protein and helps, like avocado, to feel fuller for longer. Vegetable soups and bone broth are particularly effective for interrupting a prolonged fast, but they are light lunches rich in nutrients suitable for interrupting any type of fasting (Axe, 2019). If you need to break your fast while away from home, make sure you are prepared. Prepare lunch at home the night before or make sure you can buy something healthy if necessary. Sandwiches are a good choice. Try using whole wheat bread or a piadina and include a source of protein in it. Get used to not using butter or margarine as an ingredient in your sandwich if it is already very tasty or moist. It would only serve to add saturated fats that would increase the caloric intake.

We tend to spread bread with the ugly out of habit, but if you have already used another spreadable sauce or there is a moist ingredient, you wouldn't even notice the absence of butter. The following are some healthy ideas to use as a filling to break your fast:

Boiled egg salad: boiled egg is a particularly good source of protein. You can add a little mayonnaise and some tomato or cucumber.

Roast chicken and avocado: This is a great combination of protein and unsaturated fats that will make you feel fuller for longer. If you're making roast chicken for dinner, save some for later in the week to enjoy this sandwich.

Tuna salad: choose canned tuna in a natural way to avoid extra oil and add some onion, tomato, and cucumber. The wet side brought by tuna and cucumber replaces mayonnaise or any other sauce that would only make you take in more calories than you need.

Steak: The leftovers from the dinner the night before is a fantastic and hearty filling for a sandwich with a little mustard on the bread.

Grilled vegetables: this is something you can prepare in large quantities at home and keep it in the fridge for a few days, to eat as a side dish or as a filling in sandwiches. Grill some peppers, tomatoes, onions, carrots and add some garlic and other spices if you like. They can be eaten cold in a sandwich with a slice of cheese as a source of protein.

Hummus: this chickpea sauce is just as good on bread as on piadina. It is also very nutritious.

Pork: we all love classic ham and cheese sandwiches, but processed meat is very unhealthy, and it is better to prepare some pork at home and use it as a filling for a sandwich. Pork is excellent with avocado and a little parsley.

The best options for the main meal

Pasta has a bad reputation, just like fat, but in intermittent fasting, it is one of the best dishes in terms of energy release. As with everything, quality is important, it is the pasta bought ready is not the best choice. It is always better to prepare it at home. If you eat a good pasta dish as a last meal before your next fast, your blood sugar levels stay high and you feel fuller for longer. The best thing about pasta is its versatility. You can dress it with whatever you like without any problems. The ideal would be to dress it with vegetables, garlic, and a source of protein to make your dish balanced and substantial. The ideal main meal is a portion of protein, including chicken, turkey, lamb, beef, lentils, or other legumes; two portions of vegetables (green leafy vegetables and cruciferous vegetables are great); and a source of carbohydrates that can come from potatoes, corn, or sweet potatoes. The portion of vegetables should always be double that of protein and carbohydrates. If you follow this formula and make sure you don't eat more than necessary, you will be able to have a balanced and healthy diet. If you can eat in a balanced way, you do not need supplements, but some nutrients are more difficult to take with your diet once after a certain age, for example, we need more calcium, and instead of risking being deficient and having brittle bones, it is better to take it through supplements. A slow cooking pot or a terracotta pot are useful tools for intermittent fasting because they give you the opportunity to assemble your dishes in the morning, including a source of protein and many vegetables, and cook them over low heat for the rest of the day. When you're ready to eat your main meal, you'll have dinner ready. The risk with intermittent fasting, if you are trying to lose weight, is that towards the end of the fast, your brain starts to tell you that you are very hungry. This, of course, is only in your head because you are probably no hungrier than you were before at another time of fasting, it is only your brain that tells you otherwise. This fake urgent need to eat could lead you to consume too many calories if you have not already prepared yourself properly in advance. Always make sure you have healthy, low-calorie snacks to enjoy while preparing your main meal. You can eat carrots, for example. Planning everything is the key to staying consistent, as is understanding that what your mind tells you is not always the truth. You can also prepare your own meals when you have some time to make your life easier. If you are cutting two carrots and you have time, cut them all. Using frozen vegetables is the same as using fresh vegetables in terms of nutrient content, and it's easier to keep the vegetables without worrying about them going bad. As part of your weekly programming on how to manage intermittent fasting, you can also schedule your meals to make things even easier. This way you can also see if you're eating in an overall balanced way or if you need to change something. Planning your meals in advance also makes shopping less of a chore and you're much more likely to avoid buying things you don't need. Try to avoid going shopping when you are fasting. It is well known that if we go shopping when we are hungry, we buy more food than we need and above all we buy more junk food. Try to do your weekly shopping on the day of the week when you take a break from intermittent fasting, if you have planned it, which would be ideal, or after you have already stopped fasting with a light lunch. To satisfy those who have a sweet tooth after dinner without spoiling all the progress made with a large plate of dessert, try eating a couple of squares of dark chocolate (not less than 60% cocoa), which has a much smaller impact on blood sugar levels than other desserts (Ball, n.d.). Fruit is also a good way to keep the craving for dessert at bay, so a blueberry smoothie can be great for both fasting and dessert after dinner.

Recipes suitable for Intermittent Fasting –
Light meals

The following recipes have been chosen to continue the discussion we started earlier about what foods it is best to eat to break the fast. These specific foods were chosen because they help raise blood sugar levels and keep them constant throughout the day. If there are other foods you want to try, search for their nutritional values online and enter them in an appropriate way in your diet.

Hello Hummus!

The debate about which chickpeas to choose, whether the canned chickpeas or the dry ones left to soak overnight, to make the best hummus, has existed practically since... since the invention of the canned chickpeas! Many people say that the difference is minimal in taste and it is not worth discussing about it, also because the nutritional values are the same.

Nutritional values (per portion):

Carbohydrates 12.4 g

Protein 7.5 g

Fat 5.1 g

Fibers 2.6g

Salt 0.5 g

Calories 135

Preparation time: 5 minutes

You will need: a blender

Portion per person: ¼ of the product obtained

Ingredients:

400 g of chickpeas

1 clove of garlic cut into small pieces 1 teaspoon of tahini sauce

Lemon juice

3 teaspoons Greek yogurt

Procedure:

1.Drain the chickpeas with a colander over a container to hold the liquid. Set the liquid aside.

2.In a blender pour the chickpeas, tahini sauce, lemon juice and Greek yogurt and blend until smooth.

3.Add one teaspoon of chickpeas water at a time, operating the blender after each addition, until the desired consistency is obtained.

4.To obtain a spreadable hummus, the consistency must be quite dense.

Tips & Variations:

If you want a sweeter and more pungent taste of garlic, grill it before adding it to your mix. Grilled red peppers are also an interesting addition to hummus.

Slimming smoothies

The oats in this smoothie serve to sustain blood sugar levels for a longer period to make you feel fuller for longer.

Nutritional values (per serving):

Carbohydrates 56 g

Protein 13 g

Fats 2 g

Fibers 6g

Salt 0 g

Calories 280 g

Preparation time: 5 minutes

You will need: a blender

Portion per person: 1 smoothie (all the product obtained)

Ingredients:

½ banana

1 cup of strawberries cut into pieces

¼ cup of oat flakes 1 cup of milk

¼ tablespoon of vanilla extract

½ cup of ice cubes 1 tablespoon of honey

Procedure:

1.In a blender, add the banana, strawberries, oatmeal, and milk.

2.Blend until smooth.

3.Add vanilla, ice cubes and honey and blend again until smooth.

4.If you prefer a more liquid consistency, add a little milk or water and blend again after each addition.

Tips & Variations:

Do not peel the banana before cutting it in half. This way, you can keep the half advanced for another smoothie without it blackening.

Vegetable smoothie

The intensity of the green of this smoothie makes it a very suitable option for interrupting fasting. It is rich in fiber to ensure that the rest of your day is smooth and comfortable.

Nutritional values (per serving):

Carbohydrates 27 g

Protein 7g

Fats 10 g

Fibers 6g

Salt 0.4 g

Calories 243

Preparation time: 5 minutes

You will need: a blender

Portion per person: 1 smoothie (all the product obtained)

Ingredients:

2 celery stalks 55 g spinach 100 g broccoli 1 banana

1 cup of rice milk

¼ tablespoon spirulina 4 teaspoons coconut

1 cup of water

Procedure:

1.In a blender, add the spinach, celery, and broccoli.

2.Blend until smooth.

3.Add the banana, spirulina, coconut, rice milk and water and blend again until smooth.

4.If you prefer a more liquid consistency, add a little more water or milk and blend again after each addition.

Tips & Variations:

Spirulina can be replaced with vegan protein powder.

Papaya Salad

The papaya in this delicious salad helps you digest the proteins in the peanuts, leaving you feeling full.

Nutritional values (per serving)

Carbohydrates 21 g

Protein 10 g

Fats 7 g

Fibers 7g

Salt 0.1 g

Calories 198

Preparation time: 15 minutes

You will need: no special tools Potion per person: ½ product obtained

Ingredients:

1 papaya cubed 170 g of jackdaws

170 g of soybean sprouts

A handful of unsalted peanuts Fresh basil in pieces

Fresh mint in pieces Juice of 1 lime

Procedure:

1In a large pan, over high heat, cook the jackdaws and soybean sprouts with a tablespoon of water.

2.   Fry them in the pan for 3 minutes or until they soften.

3Remove the jackdaws and soybean sprouts and pour them into a large salad bowl.

4.Add the papaya and lime juice and turn.

5.Spread basil, mint and peanuts on the salad and serve immediately.

Tips & Variations:

Salads like these can be modified as you wish. You can use nuts instead of peanuts for extra protein or use other herbs instead of basil and mint.

Delicious with fruit and nuts

The oats in this dish sustain blood sugar levels for a longer time and nuts are a source of protein that in turn help you feel fuller for longer.

Nutritional values (per serving):

Carbohydrates 35 g

Protein 15 g

Greases 11 g

Fibers 7g

Salt 0.1 g

Calories 316

Preparation time: 10 minutes

You will need: a non-stick frying pan

Portion per person: ½ product obtained

Ingredients:

55 g of mix of raisins, seeds, nuts, and goji berries 6 teaspoons of oat flakes

2 oranges

100 g Greek yogurt 1 ¾ cup water

Procedure:

1.Peel and cut the oranges and set them aside.

2.Cook the oat flakes with water in a non-stick pan for about 4 minutes or until they are cooked and thickened.

3.Divide the oats into two bowls, pour the yogurt over them and spread the chopped oranges, walnuts, raisins, seeds, and goji berries.

Tips & Variations:

Use any seasonal fruit or some fruit you prefer instead of oranges.

Avocado salad sandwich

This dish takes the unsaturated fats from the avocado and the energy from the carbohydrates in the bread to allow you to arrive full at your next meal. Tomatoes are an excellent source of antioxidants.

Nutritional values (per serving):

Carbohydrates 30 g

Protein 7g

Fats 21 g

Fibers 6g

Salt 0.9 g

Calories 332

Preparation time: 20 minutes

You will need: no special tools Portion per person: ¼ of the total product obtained Ingredients:

1 mature avocado

170 g of bread (preferably ciabatta or baguette) 500 g of cherry tomatoes

1 clove of crushed garlic 1 ½ tablespoon capers

1 small red onion sliced A handful of fresh basil

2 teaspoons of red wine vinegar

4 teaspoons of extra virgin olive oil Spices to taste

Procedure:

1.Cut the tomatoes in half and pour them in a bowl. Season according to your taste and add the avocado, onion, capers, and garlic. Mix well and leave to rest for 10 minutes; this gives the flavors the possibility to mix.

2.Cut the bread into 3 cm squares and place them on a plate. Pour half oil and half red wine vinegar on the bread. Use the spices to taste.

3.Pour the cherry tomato mix on the bread and mix slowly. Also add the basil with the rest of the extra virgin olive oil and red wine vinegar. Serve immediately.

Suggestions & Variations:

The cherry tomatoes are not essential to the realization of this dish. You can use the classic salad tomatoes and cut them into small pieces.

Slow cooking bone stock

This bone broth can be prepared overnight in a slow-cooked pot or an earthenware pot. Slow cooking is essential for this broth because it brings out the plethora of vitamins, nutrients, and minerals in the bones without destroying any of them. From this recipe you get four portions that you can keep in the fridge or freeze and then eat them on other days. The more you cook the broth, the darker it becomes. If you have animals in the house, this bone broth is also great for them!

Nutritional values (per portion):

Carbohydrates 4 g

Protein 6 g

Fats 0.3 g

Fibers 0.2g

Salt 0.65 g

Calories 45

Preparation time: 18 - 36 hours

You will need: a slow cooking pot or a terracotta pot

Portion per person: ¼ of the product obtained

Ingredients:

Chicken, veal, or beef bones 1 celery stalk

2 carrots cut into pieces 1 leek

1 bay leaf

The juice of 1 lemon

Water to fill the pot

Procedure:

1.Heat the oven to 180°C.

2.On a baking tray, spread the bones and let them cook for one hour. Turn them halfway through cooking.

3.In the meantime, peel and cut the vegetables and put them in the slow cooking pot with the bay leaf and lemon juice.

4.When the bones are ready, pour them over the vegetables in the slow cooker.

5.Fill the pot up to about 1 cm from the edge. Cover and cook for 18 - 36 hours.

6.At the end of cooking, place a sieve over a bowl and pour in the broth. Once

Remove all the bones, put the broth back into the slow cooking pot.

7.Drain the entire contents of the slow cooker to remove all solid parts.

8. Allow to cool and remove the fat that has formed on top.

Tips & Variations:

Use relatively large bones to facilitate the removal process.

Vegetable Soup

The potatoes and other tubers in this colorful dish give you enough energy until the next meal and are rich in nutrients.

Nutritional values (per serving):

Carbohydrates Protein

Fats 16 g

7 g

4 g

Fibers 0.2g

Salt 0.5 g

Calories 127

Preparation time: 25 minutes

You will need: no special tools Portion per person: ⅙ of the product obtained Ingredients:

1 large potato

1 handful of green onions 115 g spinach

255 g frozen peas

4 ¼ cup vegetable broth 1 ¼ cup white yogurt

1 clove of crushed garlic

Mint, basil, or watercress leaves to serve

Procedure:

1.Bring the vegetable stock, potato, and garlic to the boil in a pot.

2.As soon as it starts to boil, lower the heat, cover with a lid, and leave to cook for 15 minutes or until the potato becomes soft.

3.Add the frozen peas and leave to cook. Remove about four tablespoons of peas from the pot and set them aside for later use as decoration.

4.Turn off the heat and add the white yogurt and spinach, stirring everything.

5.Blend the soup with an immersion blender until smooth and season to your taste.

6.After pouring the soup into the plates, add the peas as decoration and some herbs or spices of your choice.

Tips & Variations:

This soup is already very tasty, but if you want to add more carbohydrates, you can enjoy it with a slice of crispy bread.

Beef salad

The potatoes and other tubers in this colorful dish give you enough energy until the next meal and are rich in nutrients.

Nutritional values (per serving):

Carbohydrates 7 g

Protein 21 g

Fats 17 g

Fibers 6g

Salt 0.4 g

Calories 281

Preparation time: 25 minutes (plus one hour to rest)

You will need: a barbecue

Portion per person: ⅙ product obtained

Ingredients:

2 x 250 g sirloin fillet 2 tablespoons of sesame oil

1 tablespoon low salt soy sauce 1 chilli pepper cut into pieces

2 finely chopped chilli peppers 15 g of ginger finely chopped 1 clove of garlic

The juice of 2 files

4 lettuce heads 12 radishes

3 spring onions

1 avocado well mature

½ tablespoon sesame seeds 3 carrots

½ cucumber

Procedure:

1.Remove the steaks from the refrigerator at least one hour before cooking to reach room temperature.

2.To prepare the salad sauce, mix the garlic, lime juice, finely chopped ginger, oil, soy sauce and diced chili peppers and leave the obtained product aside.

3.Cook the steaks on the barbecue for 3 minutes on the side. Leave to rest for 5 minutes after cooking and before cutting them.

4.Cut the lettuce, radishes, carrots, spring onions, avocado and cucumber and arrange them on a plate.

5.Cut the steaks and place the pieces on the freshly arranged vegetables on a plate.

6.Garnish with the sauce, sesame seeds and chili pepper.

7.Serve immediately.

Tips & Variations:

The taste of meat cooked on the barbecue is even better in this salad, but if you don't have one, you can cook it on the grill.

Recipes suitable for Intermittent Fasting for the Main Meal

To prepare a main meal suitable for intermittent fasting, you need to make sure that your energy intake will be able to sustain you until the end of the next fast the next day. Your metabolism slows down when you sleep so you should not eat your main meal less than 2 hours before going to sleep. The recipes we have chosen to share with you are suitable for the whole family and you can share them with them at dinner. They also have the benefit of being suitable for intermittent fasting.

Salmon Pasta

Pasta is a fantastic source of slow-release energy. Coupled with wild caught salmon, it becomes a great dish for the brain and a healthy source of protein. It has a high fat content but is unsaturated (good) fat from salmon.

Nutritional values (per serving):

Carbohydrates 77 g

Protein 42 g

Fats 25 g

Fibers 4g

Salt 0.21 g

Calories 682

Preparation time: 25 minutes

You will need: one non-stick frying pan Portion per person: ½ product obtained Ingredients:

200 g of tagliatelle 2 salmon fillets 100 g of arugula

2 teaspoons of creme fraiche

1 tablespoon extra-virgin olive oil Peel of 1 lemon

Procedure:

1.Heat a non-stick pan over high heat with a tablespoon of extra virgin olive oil. Place the salmon fillets on the oil in the non-stick pan and fry for 5 minutes on one side, turn on the other side and fry for another 4 minutes.

2.Remove the salmon from the pan, let it cool and then remove the skin. Cut the salmon into pieces and set it aside for the moment.

3.In another pan, cook the pasta al dente. Set aside a glass of cooking water, drain the pasta, and put it back into the pot.

4.Add the chopped salmon, arugula, creme fraiche, lemon zest to the pasta and use the remaining cooking water to stir. Turn well, being careful not to crush the salmon too much.

Suggestions & Variations:

Tagliatelle are the most suitable pasta for this dish, but you can use any other type of pasta.

Chicken Balti

Chicken is one of the best sources of animal protein. By removing the skin, you can further reduce the fat content.

Nutritional values (per serving):

Carbohydrates 31 g

Protein 40 g

Fats 6 g

Fibers 9g

Salt 0.6 g

Calories 341

Preparation time: 60 minutes

You will need: a large enough non-stick frying pan

Portion per person: ½ product obtained

Ingredients:

4 chicken legs without skin and without bones 1 onion

1 yellow bell pepper

1 red bell pepper 2 garlic cloves

225 g canned tomatoes

3 teaspoons finely chopped parsley Other parsley for garnish

⅔ cup of white yogurt

1 tablespoon of curry powder 1 tablespoon of cornstarch

Black pepper

Extra virgin olive oil for frying 2 tablespoons of cold water

100 g of water

Procedure:

1.Heat the oil in a large non-stick pan over medium heat and add the finely chopped onions.

2.Remove visible fat from chicken legs and cut them into four pieces each. Season with black pepper.

3.Add the peppers and chopped chicken to the pan with the onion and cook for 3 minutes, turning the chicken pieces from time to time.

4.In a bowl, mix the cornstarch with two tablespoons of water and add the yogurt. Stir well.

5.Add the garlic and curry powder into the pan with the chicken and cook for 30 seconds.

 6.Add the yogurt mixture, 100 grams of water, parsley and canned tomatoes into the pan and bring to the boil. Cook for 25 minutes until the chicken is fully cooked and the sauce has thickened.

7.Season with black pepper and a little parsley.

Tips & Variations:

This recipe can also be made by replacing chicken with turkey. Serve this way or add a carbohydrate source of your choice.

Spaghetti Bolognese without meat

This vegetarian dish is rich in vegetable proteins.

Nutritional values (per serving):

Carbohydrates 61 g

Protein 19 g

Fats 15 g

Fibers 19 g

Salt 0.4 g

Calories 494

Preparation time: 45 minutes

You will need: no special tools Portion per person: ¼ product obtained Ingredients:

425 g of lentils

225 g of wholemeal pasta

30 g of dehydrated porcini mushrooms 1 diced onion

1 carrot diced 1 leek

1 celery stalk 2 cloves of garlic

¼ cup of extra virgin olive oil Salt and pepper for seasoning

1 bay leaf

½ teaspoon of oregano

½ teaspoon of basil

½ teaspoon of thyme

¼ cup of almond milk

425 g of canned tomatoes with sauce 2 teaspoons of pomdoro concentrate Parmesan cheese for dressing

Procedure:

1.Soak the dehydrated porcini mushrooms in hot water for 15 minutes. Remove them once rehydrated and dry them with paper towels. Finely cut the porcini mushrooms.

2.Dice the celery, leek, carrot, onion, and garlic and mix them together.

3.Heat the extra virgin olive oil in a pan over medium heat and add the onion and mushroom mixture and cook for 8 minutes or until the vegetables are cooked.

4.Add the almond milk, bay leaf, spices and lentils and cook for about 3 minutes stirring occasionally.

5.When the liquid in the pan has almost completely evaporated, add the canned tomatoes and tomato paste.

6.Mix everything well and continue to cook for another 10 minutes, stirring continuously to prevent it from sticking to the bottom of the pan.

7.Remove the bay leaf and season the pasta with the sauce obtained.

Serve with garlic bread or a salad.

Steak with sweet potatoes

Although it is not the case to eat too much red meat, if it is something you like to eat, occasionally it is fine. The important thing is that the portion is small and is accompanied by healthy side dishes.

Nutritional values (per portion):

Carbohydrates 43 g

Protein 33 g

Fats 0.5 g

Fibers 12g

Salt 0.4 g

Calories 452

Preparation time: 35 minutes

You will need: no special tools

Portion per person: ½ product obtained

Ingredients:

2 x 125 g of steak 255 g of sweet potatoes 200 g of spinach

2 onions

1 green bell pepper 85 g cherry tomatoes

3 teaspoons of extra virgin olive oil 1 tablespoon of thyme

1 teaspoon of paprika 2 cloves of garlic

1 tablespoon of tomato paste 140 g of water

Procedure:

1. Preheat the oven to 240°C

2. Peel the sweet potatoes and cut them into slices. Put them in a bowl with two tablespoons of oil and thyme. Mix well.

3. Place the sweet potatoes in a baking tray and set aside for the moment.

4. Heat a tablespoon of oil in a non-stick pan. Add the onions, cover with a lid, and leave to cook until transparent (about 5 minutes). Add the green bell pepper and garlic and cook for another 5 minutes.

5. Put the sweet potatoes in the oven and cook for 15 minutes.

6. Add the paprika and water to the pan with the onions and stir. Add the tomato paste and the cherry tomatoes. Cover and cook for 10 minutes.

7. Cover the steaks with a little oil. Fry in a pan for about 3 minutes on each side. Leave to rest for 5 minutes.

8. Cook the spinach quickly in a pan or microwave.

9. Place everything and add the sauce on the steaks with the spinach and sweet potatoes as a side dish.

Tips & Variations:

Choose any type of meat cut, but always try to choose a low-fat one to keep the saturated fat away as much as possible.

Mexican Pasta

You only need a small portion of this dish to satiate yourself because both the pasta and the avocado release a lot of energy.

Nutritional values (per serving):

Carbohydrates 65 g

Protein 15 g

 Fats 15 g

Fibers 18g

Salt 0.4 g

Calories 495

Preparation time: 30 minutes

You will need: no special tools Portion per person: ½ product obtained Ingredients:

100 g of wholemeal penne 1 avocado

1 onion

2 garlic cloves 1 yellow bell pepper

400 g canned tomatoes 200 g corn kernels

Peel and juice of half a lime A handful of parsley Additional parsley for garnish

1 tablespoon of extra virgin olive oil

2 teaspoons of finely chopped chili pepper

½ tablespoon of cumin seeds

1 tablespoon parsley finely chopped 1 teaspoon onion finely chopped

Procedure:

1.Cook the pasta al dente.

2.Heat the oil in a pan over medium heat and fry the bell pepper and onion until it becomes transparent. Add the garlic, tomatoes, spices, corn, and half of the water in the corn can.

3.Cook for 15 minutes.

4.Sprinkle lemon juice on the avocado and mix with finely chopped onion.

5.Drain the penne and add them to the sauce, adding parsley.

6.Place and add the avocado. Garnish with more parsley.

Tips & Variations:

If you prefer it a little hotter, add some finely chopped fresh chili pepper to the avocado mix.

Spicy soup with chickpeas and lentils

Both chickpeas and lentils in this delicious soup are great sources of energy and will help you feel full for a long time. This soup can also be frozen so you can make more, freeze it, and eat it after lunch or dinner without having to cook.

Nutritional values (per serving):

Carbohydrates 17.2 g

Protein 8.5 g

Fat 2.4 g

Fibers 6.1g

Salt 0.4 g

Calories 136

Preparation time: 40 minutes

You will need: an electric pressure cooker

Portion per person: one bowl

Ingredients:

1 cup of lentils

1 cup of dried chickpeas soaked overnight 1 onion

2 celery stalks

400 g canned tomatoes 2 glasses of chicken broth 2 teaspoons of lime juice

425 g pumpkin cut into pieces

½ tablespoon dried chili pepper 3 cups water

½ cup of coriander finely chopped 2 tablespoons of extra virgin olive oil 3 cloves of garlic

2 teaspoons of paprika 4 g of fresh ginger

1 tablespoon of cumin powder

1 tablespoon coriander powder

Procedure:

1.Drain the remaining chickpeas overnight and rinse them with cold water.

2.Heat the oil in a pressure cooker and cook the onion, garlic and grated ginger until the onions become soft.

3.Add the coriander, cumin powder, paprika and dried chili pepper and cook for a few minutes.

4.Add the water, chicken stock, tomatoes, and chickpeas. Close the pressure cooker tightly and set the cooking to "high pressure" for 25 minutes.

5.Reduce the pressure after 25 minutes and remove the lid carefully and keep the steam away from your face.

6.Add the lentils, pumpkin, celery, and cover with the lid again.

7.Bring the cooking under high pressure and cook for 5 minutes. Decrease the pressure and cook for another 5 minutes. Add the lime juice and fresh coriander.

If you don't have a pressure cooker, you can cook this soup in a slow cooking pot or on a normal stove. Cook until the chickpeas and lentils are soft. It is not necessary to blend the soup to make it liquid.

Lamb stew

Lamb is one of the healthiest red meats and can be eaten in stews and curries.

Nutritional values (per portion):

Carbohydrates

Protein 31.2 g

34 g

Fats 21.9 g

Fibers 9.6g

Salt 0.4 g

Calories 477

Preparation time: 95 minutes

You will need: no special tools Portion per person: ¼ product obtained Ingredients:

4 cuts of lamb neck 1 onion

2 garlic cloves

400 g canned tomatoes

½ cup of water 8 spring onions

350 g baby carrots

1 cup frozen peas

2 teaspoons of smooth-leaf parsley 1 tablespoon of extra virgin olive oil
450 g new potatoes

Procedure:

1. Heat the extra virgin olive oil in a pot over medium heat. Leave the lamb to brown. The more you brown it well, the more flavor you will get. Obviously, you don't have to burn the meat, but this process also helps to melt the remaining fat in the lamb.

2. When the lamb is cooked, remove it from the pan and cook the onion and garlic until the onion appears transparent. Add the lamb again accompanied by tomatoes and water. Leave to boil for 30 - 45 minutes with the lid on. Turn from time to time taking care not to further break up the ingredients.

3. When the meat starts to soften, add the new potatoes, spring onions and baby carrots. Cook for 15 minutes or until the potatoes and carrots are soft.

4. Add the peas and cook until ready. Season according to your taste and add parsley during the planting.

Tips & Variations:

The lamb needs time to soften and therefore this is not a dish that can be cooked in a casserole because the other ingredients would become too soft and the meat would remain harder. Lamb fat is one of the healthiest forms of animal fat, but in such a dish it is best to cut it off before cooking.

Braised pork with chili

This dish has a low carbohydrate and high protein content and is perfect for those who want to lose weight or tone muscles and increase muscle mass.

Nutritional values (per serving):

Carbohydrates 8.1 g

Protein 44.6 g

Fats 26 g

Fibers 2g

Salt 0.5 g

Calories 447

Preparation time: 60 minutes

You will need: kitchen string

Portion per person: ¼ product obtained

Ingredients:

680 g of pork shoulder without bones 4 cloves of garlic

4 anchovy fillets

400 g canned tomatoes 1 cup water

2 tablespoons of extra virgin olive oil 2 teaspoons of fresh oregano

1 tablespoon capers

½ tablespoon dried chili pepper

½ cup of black olives

Procedure:

1.Wrap the pork shoulder and tie it with kitchen string at 2 cm intervals to keep the meat together.

2.Heat a pan large enough and brown the shoulder of pork to join the meat. When it is done browning, remove the meat and set it aside.

3.Heat some oil in the pan and cook the garlic and anchovies, stirring occasionally. Add the tomatoes, water, oregano, chili pepper and capers. Add the pork and cook for 40 minutes. When the pig is still slightly pink but soft, remove it from the pan. If you prefer to cook it more, leave it on the fire for another 5 minutes. Once removed from the pan, let it rest for 5 minutes before removing the kitchen string and then cut it. This allows the fibres of the meat to stay together so that you can cut slices more easily and cleanly.

4.Add the olives to the sauce and season according to your taste. Serve the pork shoulder slices on a bed of polenta covered with the sauce just prepared.

Suggestions & Variations:

Instead of polenta, you can serve this dish with a slice of crispy bread.

Chicken with butter

Chicken with butter is a light and delicate dish of incredibly famous Indian origin and is suitable for the whole family and its source of lean protein also makes it a healthy dish.

Nutritional values (per serving):

Carbohydrates 23.5 g

Protein 48.7 g

Fats 58.1 g

Fibers 4g

Salt 0.5 g

Calories 814

Preparation time: 60 minutes

You will need: no special tools Portion per person: ¼ product obtained Ingredients:

4 chicken breasts

1 tablespoon of lemon juice

½ cup of white yogurt

A piece of 5 cm ginger grated 2 tablespoons of garam masala

1 tablespoon seed oil 40 g butter

1 onion

4 cloves of garlic

1 tablespoon coriander powder 1 tablespoon cumin powder

1 tablespoon of cinnamon powder 1 tablespoon of paprika

2 tablespoons of tomato paste 400 g of tomato puree

Chicken broth

2 teaspoons of honey

⅓ cup of cream

½ cup fresh coriander

Procedure:

1.Mix the chicken, lemon juice, grated ginger, yogurt and garam masala in a large enough bowl. Make sure the chicken is well marinated.

2.Heat half oil and half butter in a large pot and brown the marinated chicken. Remove from the pot and set aside.

3.Heat the remaining oil and butter and cook the onion and garlic until the onion becomes soft.

4.Put the chicken back into the pot with the tomato paste, tomato puree, chicken broth and honey. Cook for 30 minutes or until the chicken is cooked.

5.Add the cooking cream and season to taste.

6.Place and serve with fresh coriander.

Tips & Variations:

Serve with a starch to taste. You can increase the taste of this dish by adding more garam masala.

Conclusion

As women over 50, we know we must expect health problems with aging. We see our friends and family gain weight, have menopausal symptoms and another long list of non-contagious diseases such as diabetes and hypertension. We enter this period of our lives with a sense of trepidation, we feel that we are not in control and our body becomes an enemy. The reality, however, is extremely far from the truth. There are certainly some health problems that we must be careful about, but our 50 years and later could be the period of our life when we show more vitality, because we no longer must focus our energies on others and therefore, we have more time to think about our needs and achieve our goals. This, in fact, should be an exciting time for us, and if we can learn how to make it so and learn what is going on inside our bodies, it can really be. There is no better opportunity to take our physical and mental health where we want it than when we reach our 50th birthday. Intermittent fasting is one of the most holistic methods of doing this. By following a simple and well-structured plan that tells us how to eat, we can counteract the effects of aging, lose weight, reduce, and sometimes even eliminate certain diseases and increase our longevity. Through intermittent fasting, instead of seeing our body as an enemy working against us, we use it to our advantage by exploiting its natural processes.

We have much more control over our bodies than we think. The key is to understand how our body works. At this age, many of us have tried many diets and realized that most of them are more harmful than anything else. The flexibility of intermittent fasting means that we can match our lifestyles perfectly and not the other way around. Most food programs that aim to help you lose weight fail because they are too difficult to follow in the long term or because the foods you need are too expensive. Intermittent fasting doesn't dictate what you eat, and you choose when to do it. If you maintain a healthy diet, you can indulge in your favorite foods from time to time without feeling like you're failing. It's this flexibility, coupled with the idea that you're not "forcing yourself" to make intermittent fasting probably the easiest diet to follow. When you start intermittent fasting and explain to others what you are doing, you need to prepare yourself for some doubts or misunderstandings that others may have. People generally see fasting as something strange and may wonder why you would do such a "terrible" thing to yourself. You can handle this kind of situation in two ways. You can explain to them that you have learned in this book to make them understand the world of intermittent fasting too, or you can smile at them and tell them that they don't need to worry about you because you will be fine. The former, of course, might be more useful to them because they might even decide to start on the same path as you, but not everyone is open-minded enough to accept that what they have been taught about food all their lives are largely wrong. Suffice it to say that when they begin to see your improvements, they will also be more open to intermittent fasting. Fasting is a centuries-old practice. If the diets that have emerged in recent years make you skeptical, you are not alone. Many of these trendy diets have extraordinarily little scientific basis to support them. They have also only been practiced for a few years so there is little evidence of their long-term effects on our bodies. Although this may not seem like a noteworthy problem for a 20-year-old person, as they get older, we need to make sure that what we do to be healthy has a scientific basis. Fortunately, intermittent fasting has a lot of scientific research behind it as well as a lot of testimonies that tell us the results obtained by people who have tried it. Fasting works perfectly with the processes of our body; it improves and stabilizes them. Fasting does not only help us to lose weight; it has benefits on our whole body and on a cognitive and emotional level. Although there are some side effects in the first few days of fasting, none of them are permanent or insurmountable and with a little preparation they can be overcome very easily and quickly. The negative effects last for a short time and your body can easily adapt to what are its natural processes. Our bodies are not really made to eat constantly, and from an evolutionary point of view, we are much closer to the fasting regime than to eating constantly. This is demonstrated by the fact that fasting triggers a series of beneficial processes that occur naturally when we fast. Food is important from the point of view of nutrients and is also enjoyable to eat, but our society has turned food into our enemy rather than an ally. If you consider the fact that only 20 years ago the World Health Organization's focus was on malnutrition and starvation, while in 2019 they started to focus on obesity and overnutrition, this shows exactly how wrong our relationship with food has become. The World Health Organization has even coined a new term to describe how we eat today; it is called the Western Diet. The term is not a compliment because it highlights a diet based primarily on convenience foods, high sugar levels and excessive consumption of red meat. The Western Diet is not only a problem in the United States. With the spread of advertising around the world, it is becoming popular in many countries, and studies show a negative change even in countries where previously the diet was generally quite healthy. Alcohol has also become a huge health problem, and many women over 40 have abdominal fat problems due to high sugar alcohol drinks. Although there is no need to avoid alcohol completely, the intake should be minimized, especially as we get older because it has an even stronger impact on our body. Overnutrition is just as dangerous as malnutrition and is one of the main causes of non-contagious diseases. As we get older, we can start caring about our bodies and treating them better than we have ever done in the past. Keep in mind that you don't need to change the lifestyle of your entire family in order to change yours. Fasting fits perfectly in our lives as they are, so there is no need for the other members of your family to make changes as well.

By fasting, you not only ensure a better life for yourself, but you also ensure it for your family. You will have more energy, live longer, and have a better quality of life when you spend time with loved ones. Only for this reason it is worth it. A healthy diet includes lots of fruits and vegetables, lean proteins (preferably vegetable or very lean if animal), unsaturated fats and lots of fiber. Highly processed foods with a high level of sodium and saturated fats are not good for any food plan. Including fresh fruits and vegetables in your diet raises antioxidant levels and when this is accompanied by the natural benefits of autophagy, it has additional benefits for a longer life. In Intermittent Fasting for Women Over 50, we've given you all the information you need to make fasting an integral part of your lifestyle. Our recommended foods can be adapted to your needs as well as the recipes we have provided you with. Using the general ideas, we have given you, you can look for other resources from which to take new recipes. In the field of food choices, the key is balance. You don't have to deny yourself something you really like just because it contains a few calories. Food is yes useful to support our bodily processes, but it is also enjoyment, and there is no need to limit ourselves so much that we think that instead of living we barely exist and are not enjoying life. It is undeniable that when we socialize, food is a fundamental part of that pleasure, and it is not a bad thing. The important thing is not to overdo it with food or use the holidays as an excuse to eat too much and there will be no problem associating food with being social. Fasting should add to your life and never take away, so if you feel that it is too much for you or that after a few months you still hate it, then you should review the way you are doing it. Often, with just a small change such as slightly decreasing the fasting window or changing the time when it must happen, we can completely revolutionize our experience with intermittent fasting. The idea is to achieve your weight goal while enjoying increased energy, vitality, and overall well-being. Getting into your 40s should not be a time of difficulty or trepidation, and intermittent fasting as a lifestyle is the key to making sure you are living life properly from all points of view.

REFERENCES

6 Popular Ways to Do Intermittent Fasting. (2017). Healthline. https://www.healthline.com/nutrition/6-ways-to-do-intermittent-fasting

11 High-Energy Foods for Intermittent Fasting. (n.d.). Food Network. Retrieved February 21, 2020, from https://www.foodnetwork.com/healthyeats/diets/2019/07/high-energy-foods- intermittent fasting

Fung, J. (2019, April 25). Diet Doctor. Diet Doctor. https://www.dietdoctor.com/intermittent- fasting

Gunnars, K. (2017, June 4). What Is Intermittent Fasting? Explained in Human Terms. Healthline; Healthline Media. https://www.healthline.com/nutrition/what-is-intermittent-fasting#section2

What an Intermittent Fasting and a Healthy Diet Boost Mental Health. (2019, May 1). 24Life. https://www.24life.com/how-intermittent-fasting-and-a-healthy-diet-boost-mental-health/

I Went into Early Perimenopause & Learned Why Balancing Blood Sugar Is So Important. (2019, January 30). Mindbodygreen. https://www.mindbodygreen.com/articles/blood-sugar-and-perimenopause

Jeanie Lerche Davis. (2007, March 23). Get-Fit Advice for Women Over 50. WebMD; WebMD. https://www.webmd.com/women/guide/women-over-50-fitness-tips

Kresser, C. (2019, March 25). Intermittent Fasting: The Science Behind the Trend. Chris Kresser; chriskresser.com. https://chriskresser.com/intermittent-fasting-the-science-behind-the-trend/

Pawlowski, A. (2019, January 16). How to lose weight with intermittent fasting, 16:8 diet. TODAY.Com; TODAY. https://www.today.com/health/how-lose-weight-intermittent-fasting-

16-8-diet-t132608

Practical   tips   for   fasting. (2016,   September   15).
          Diet   Doctor. https://www.dietdoctor.com/practical-tips-
fasting

What Foods Are Best to Eat on an Intermittent Fasting Diet? (n.d.).
Greatist. Retrieved February 21, 2020, from
https://greatist.com/eat/what-to-eat-on-an-intermittent-fasting-diet#1

CPSIA information can be obtained
at www.ICGtesting.com
Printed in the USA
LVHW060318290321
682791LV00013B/998